Intermittent Fasting for Women Over 50

The Top 7 Rules to Delay Aging and Rejuvenate Yourself in 4 Weeks. Find Out How to Burn Belly Fat and Maintain Hormonal Balance.

Bonus: 21-Days Meal Plan

Tayler kimberlyn

© **Copyright 2021 by Tayler kimberlyn - All rights reserved.**

The content contained within this book may not be reproduced, duplicated or transmitted without direct written permission from the author or the publisher.

Under no circumstances will any blame or legal responsibility be held against the publisher, or author, for any damages, reparation, or monetary loss due to the information contained within this book. Either directly or indirectly.

Legal Notice:

This book is copyright protected. This book is only for personal use. You cannot amend, distribute, sell, use, quote or paraphrase any part, or the content within this book, without the consent of the author or publisher.

Disclaimer Notice:

Please note the information contained within this document is for educational and entertainment purposes only. All effort has been executed to present accurate, up to date, and reliable, complete information. No warranties of any kind are declared or implied. Readers acknowledge that the author is not engaging in the rendering of legal, financial, medical or professional advice. The content within this book has been derived from various sources. Please consult a licensed professional before attempting any techniques outlined in this book.

By reading this document, the reader agrees that under no circumstances is the author responsible for any losses, direct or indirect, which are incurred as a result of the use of information contained within this document, including, but not limited to, - errors, omissions, or inaccuracies.

Table of Contents

Introduction 1
Part One Chapter 1: What Is If? 2
   How Intermittent Fasting Works 2
Chapter 2: Why Start If, Advantages And Disadvantages 4
   The Advantages Of Intermittent Fasting for Women Over 50 6
   Is Intermittent Fasting Healthy For Diabetics? 8
   Intermittent Fasting And Your Menstrual Cycle. 12
Chapter 3: Types Of If 14
   Types Of Intermittent Fasting 15
Chapter 4: Food To Eat And To Avoid 17
Chapter 5: Super Foods To Eat For Woman Over 50 20
Chapter 6: Mistakes To Avoid During If 23
Chapter 7: Autophagy Of If 26
   All You Need To Know About Autophagy 27
Chapter 8: Manage Menopause 30
   Menopause Natural Treatments That Actually Work 31
   How To Lose Weight During Menopause 34
Chapter 9: The Rules To Slow Down Aging And Rejuvenate In 4 Weeks 38
   Slow The Aging Process-In 7 Days 42
   How To Age Well 46
Chapter 10: Exercises To Do With The If 52
   Essential Guide 54
   Workouts And Intermittent Fasting 57
   How To Lose Belly Fat While Maintaining Normal Hormonal Balance 59
Part Two Intermittent Fasting Recipes &21-Days Meal Plan 64
Breakfast, Snack, Lunch And Dinner Recipes 65
Conclusion 133

Introduction

Intermittent fasting is a concept you might be familiar with. Nowadays, it's a common topic. When looking for a way to lose weight, some people bring it up. Others speak of it as a way to boost their overall wellbeing. What is intermittent fasting, though? Is it beneficial to your health? What advantages are there? Are side effects present? Is it acceptable for all people?

Road to better health

Intermittent fasting is not a weight-loss technique. Although it may have some of the same health advantages as a diet, it just is a pattern of eating. It means you're fasting (not eating) every day for a certain period (usually an extended time). You then eat each day for another period (usually a smaller period of time). You can drink drinks that do not contain calories while fasting, including water, black coffee, and unsweetened tea.

The division of fasting and eating each day is called an eating plan. The 16:8 schedule is one of the most common and simple to follow. This means you fast for 16 hours and only eat your daily meals for 8 hours. You would want to fast from 7 p.m. to 11 a.m. the next day, for example. Around 11 a.m. and 7 p.m., you'd eat a good lunch and dinner. You're not allowed to eat anything after 7 p.m. until 11 a.m. the next day. This is just an example of how things have been in the past. You can pick either a 16-hour or 8-hour time block that fits best for your schedule. But keeping your eating window at the same every day is crucial.

18:6 fasting (fasting for 18 hours and eating for 6 hours) and alternate days are two other intermittent fasting schedules. You fast for 24 hours on alternate days, then eat a balanced diet for the next 24 hours, then fast again for the next 24 hours. Using the every-other-day format, this schedule continues. 5:2 is another schedule choice. This is when you fast for two days a week, and eat the other five days of a regular, balanced diet. This is a little different, however, because, on your fasting days, this routine requires you to eat one small meal of 500 to 600 calories.

Your eating window is the amount of time you're allowed to consume. Focus on maintaining a balanced diet and portion control during your eating window. Don't consume too many calories and stop fast food and junk food. Although you don't have to eat something specific, you can make sure you're getting enough nutrients.

PART ONE

Chapter 1: What is IF?

Intermittent fasting is a diet technique that includes eating and fasting for brief periods (meaning no food at all or very low-calorie consumption).

Fasting has been used for religious, cultural, and spiritual purposes throughout history and around the world. Fasting has become popular among those who want to lose weight without having to give up specific foods as a result of the media coverage provided to diets like the 5:2 diet in recent years.

IF focuses on the periods of time that we don't feed – what we term "fasting." The frequency and length of these fasting periods are determined by the type of diet followed and the schedule of the person. The following are some examples of common IF eating patterns:

Choosing a time frame for eating each day and abstaining from eating outside of it. The 16:8 diet, for example, includes fasting for 16 hours a day and eating within an 8-hour window. One of the most common ways to do this is to miss breakfast and eat only between noon and 8 p.m., resulting in a 16-hour fast every day (between 8pm and midday the next day). Other diet variants include 6-hour or shorter feeding times.

Selecting a normal day of the week or month to fast for a full 24-hour cycle. If you finish dinner at 8 p.m. one night, for example, you won't eat again until 8 p.m. the next day.

Choosing to consume very few calories on some days of the week while consuming a regular amount of calories the rest of the week. The 5:2 diet, for example, includes consuming just 25% of a regular calorie intake (500 kcals for women, 600 kcals for men) on two days per week and eating regularly on the remaining five.

How Intermittent Fasting Works

How your metabolic system works is affected by fasting for at least 12 hours. Your metabolic system is responsible for converting the energy you get from the foods and drinks you eat. Your body gets much of its energy from a sugar called glucose. In the foods you consume and drinks you drink, glucose is found. Since you're eating and drinking regularly while you consume three meals a day, your body maintains a constant glucose level.

When you fast for more than 12 hours, however, the glucose levels in your body tend to dip because you don't eat as much. When your body doesn't have access to the glucose it needs for energy, it turns to fat for food. As this occurs, the body's fatty acids are absorbed into your bloodstream. A chemical called ketones are formed by them. The ketones are then used by your body as its energy source. A metabolic transition is what this is referred to as. Your body is making the transition from glucose to ketones.

You can lose weight if your body uses ketones instead of fat. However, ketones can have a beneficial effect on your body's organs and cells behind the scenes.

You must fast for at least 12 hours to enjoy the benefits of intermittent fasting. That's how long it takes for your body to turn from using energy for glucose to using energy for fat. It will also take some time for the body to adapt to this new eating routine. So, don't immediately expect results. You'll likely have to wait between 2 and 4 weeks to see or experience any improvements.

Is it safe?
The fasting stage of these diets receives a lot of attention, but the food eaten during your 'eating windows' must be of high nutritional value to be a safe, reliable, and nutritious way of eating. Include essential fats such as those found in fatty fish, nuts, and seeds, as well as lean protein sources, wholegrains and starchy carbs, and plenty of fruit and vegetables to get enough dietary fiber, vitamins, and minerals.

Is it effective in terms of weight loss and is it long-term?
When comparing IF to daily calorie restriction, studies show that it is just as effective at encouraging weight loss in people who are overweight or obese. However, the results can vary based on your particular circumstances and the amount of weight you need to lose. Your ability to continue this eating style in the future will decide how successful it is in the long run. This is because IF is more of an eating regimen than a diet, so maintaining a weight loss is largely dependent on how well you adapt your eating habits over time.

What are the variations between the various versions of IF?
There are several different approaches to IF, with some being more severe than others. It's important to remember that there's still a lot we don't know about this form, such as the best fasting pattern and calorie cap. If you're thinking of following this diet, check with your doctor or a medical professional to make sure it's right for you. Many people find that a moderate fast, in which they finish all of their food by 7 p.m. and then wait until 8 a.m. the next morning to eat breakfast, is a more healthy strategy that also reaps some of the alleged benefits.

When it comes to fasting, who should be more cautious?
Fasting can be stopped if you are pregnant, breastfeeding, diabetic, or have a disorder that allows you to keep a close eye on your blood sugar levels. Furthermore, some individuals are more vulnerable to the harmful effects of fasting. Headaches and dizziness, inability to focus, flare-ups of a long-term health condition like gout, or changes in the way such drugs are processed and used by the body are all potential side effects. The elderly, the young (under 18 years of age), those on medication, those with a low body mass index (BMI), and those with emotional or psychological problems around food, including any history of eating disorders, are all vulnerable groups who should exercise caution.

Chapter 2: Why start IF, advantages and disadvantages

Intermittent fasting, the common health movement that includes not eating for specific periods of time, has many benefits and a few disadvantages, just like anything else.

Intermittent fasting improves body structure, decreases disease risk, and improves cognitive function.

Intermittent fasting has a range of disadvantages, including the fact that it can be difficult to sustain long-term, may have an impact on your social life, and may cause health problems.

It's virtually impossible to perform some sort of diet or exercise research without coming across details on intermittent fasting.

The diet trend means going without food for a fixed period of time, but one thing to bear in mind about intermittent fasting is that there are several ways to implement this form of dietary trend.

Some people suggest a 16:8 diet, in which you don't eat anything for 16 hours and then eat all of your meals and calories for the day over a fixed eight-hour cycle. Some people recommend the 5:2 diet, in which you fast and consume about 500 calories for two days, then eat whatever you want for the remaining five days of the week. Other ways of intermittent fasting propose fasting for a full 36 hours once a week.

The advantage of intermittent fasting is that it helps you to find the alternative that works best for you. And, as with anything, there are advantages and disadvantages.

Pro: Intermittent fasting helps you lose weight and boost your body composition.

Since you don't consume calories when you fast, it's fair to believe that consuming less than you usually would result in weight loss. Fasting helps you to burn out all of your stored sugars and then tap into your fat reserves for energy. We continue to lose body fat as we begin to burn fat stores.

According to Healthline, intermittent fasting enhances body composition by requiring a calorie deficit, encouraging weight loss and reduced body fat, and inducing beneficial improvements in our metabolism through its impact on hormones.

Cons: It can be difficult to maintain long-term.

Intermittent fasting involves going without food for a specified period of time, then eating a set amount of calories in a set window of time, and repeating the process to create a caloric deficit. Due to low energy, cravings, routines, and the discipline needed to stick to the particular time frames surrounding your periods of intermittent fasting, this extended period of zero-calorie intake can be difficult to stick with long-term.

Intermittent fasting is often difficult to sustain over time due to the amount of self-control necessary. Intermittent fasting can be daunting on both sides; not eating while you're supposed to be fasting and not bingeing when it's time to eat are both equally essential.

Although this may be difficult, it is necessary for the process and, in the end, reaping the benefits of intermittent fasting.

Pro: Intermittent fasting can help prevent disease and reduce the risk of disease.

Intermittent fasting has the potential to "have a beneficial effect on certain significant cardiovascular disease risk markers." Fasting can help control diabetes, lower cholesterol, and lower blood pressure in addition to weight loss, both of which are essential factors to monitor for disease prevention.

According to a study conducted by researchers at the University of Surrey, people who adopted an intermittent fasting diet had a 9 percent lower blood pressure than those who followed a more conventional, daily diet, which had a 2 percent rise.

Another research discovered that intermittent fasting increased sleep time, which decreased blood sugar and inflammation, two major contributors to chronic diseases including heart disease and diabetes.

Cons: It can affect your social life.

Let's face it, the vast majority of our social experiences take place over food and beverages. When fasting, you must either have the courage to refrain from indulging or find ways to maintain a social life without breaking your fast.

It is possible, although difficult.

Fasting, on the other hand, can be boring. Fasting causes you to have lower energy levels than normal, so you may not want to go out or feel like you need to rest to save the energy you do have.

It's a delicate juggling act.

Intermittent fasting is beneficial to brain health.

According to Mark Mattson, professor of neurology at John Hopkins University and chief of the Laboratory of Neurosciences at the National Institute on Aging, fasting increases the rate of neurogenesis in the brain, which is characterized as "the growth and development of new brain cells and nerve tissues." As a consequence, brain output, mood, concentration, and memory improve.

Mattson also believes that depriving oneself of food challenges the brain and induces it to take disease-prevention steps. This is due to the body entering ketosis, a metabolic condition in which fat is used as a fuel source to "boost energy and banish brain fog."

We've all learned that puzzles and other brain-challenging tasks are good for us, and it seems that fasting poses similar challenges.

Cons: There's a greater chance of any detrimental health effects.

Hormonal imbalances can occur in those who already lead active lifestyles or are leaner individuals before starting intermittent fasting.

This could result in abnormal menstrual cycles and the likelihood of fertility problems for people who identify as women. Hormonal imbalances can cause insomnia, elevated stress, and thyroid issues in anyone.

Intermittent fasting is usually healthy for most people when performed under the guidance or approval of a physician and with proper observation of bodily functions.

The Advantages of Intermittent Fastingfor Women Over 50

Lower metabolism, achy knees, decreased muscle mass, and even sleep problems all make it more difficult to lose weight after 50. Simultaneously, losing weight, especially dangerous belly fat, can significantly lower your risk of serious health problems including diabetes, heart attacks, and cancer.

Of course, when you grow older, the chances of contracting several diseases rise. In certain cases, intermittent fasting for women over 50 could act as a virtual fountain of youth when it comes to weight loss and minimizing the risk of developing usually age-related illnesses.

What Is the Method of Intermittent Fasting?

Intermittent fasting, also referred to as IF, won't cause you to starve yourself. It also doesn't give you a license to eat tons of unhealthy food during the time that you don't fast. Instead of eating meals and snacks all day, you eat within a specific window of time.

The majority of people stick to an IF schedule that allows them to fast for 12 to 16 hours every day. They eat healthy meals and snacks the majority of the time. Since most people sleep for around eight hours during their fasting hours, sticking to this eating window isn't as difficult as it sounds. You're also advised to drink zero-calorie beverages like water, tea, and coffee.

For the best intermittent fasting results, build an eating routine that works for you. Consider the following example:

12-hour fasts: If you follow a 12-hour fast, you can miss breakfast and eat at lunchtime. You could eat an early supper and avoid evening snacks if you prefer to eat your morning meal. A 12-12 fast is reasonably easy to manage for most older women.

16-hour fasts: A 16-8 IF schedule can yield faster results. Within 8 hours, most people prefer to eat two meals and a snack or two. For example, the eating window may be set between noon and 8 p.m., or between 8 a.m. and 4 p.m.

5-2 schedule: Limited eating times may not be ideal for you regularly. Another choice is to follow a 12- or 16-hour fast for five days and then relax for two days. For example, you might do intermittent fasting throughout the week and eat normally on the weekends.

Fasting every other day: Another choice is to eat very few calories on alternating days. For instance, you might limit your calories to under 500 calories one day and then eat normally the next. It's worth noting that regular IF fasts never necessitate calorie restrictions that low.

As for every diet, you'll get the best results if you're consistent. At the same time, on special occasions, you should take a break from this sort of eating routine. You should try various forms of intermittent fasting to see which one fits better for you. Many people begin their IF journey with the 12-12 plan and then move to the 16-8 plan. After that, try to stick to your schedule as closely as possible.

What Triggers Intermittent Fasting to Be Effective?
Some people claim that IF has helped them lose weight simply because the small eating window forces them to consume fewer calories. For example, instead of three meals and two snacks, they can only have time for two meals and one snack. They become more aware of the foods they eat and prefer to avoid refined sugars, unhealthy fats, and empty calories.

Of course, you have the right to consume whatever healthy foods you choose. While some people use intermittent fasting to minimize their total calorie consumption, some use it in combination with a keto, vegan, or other diets.

Women's Intermittent Fasting Benefits Could Go Beyond Calorie Restrictions
Although some nutritionists claim that IF only works because it allows people to eat less, others disagree. They assume that intermittent fasting outcomes are higher than conventional meal schedules with the same amount of calories and other nutrients. Studies have also proposed that fasting for several hours a day accomplishes more than just calorie restriction.

There are some metabolic changes that IF induces that could help account for synergistic benefits:

Insulin: Lower insulin levels during the fasting cycle can aid fat burning.

HGH levels increase as insulin levels fall, encouraging fat burning and muscle development.

Noradrenaline: When the nervous system senses an empty stomach, it sends this chemical to cells, instructing them to release fat for food.

Is Intermittent Fasting Beneficial to Your Health?
Is intermittent fasting a good way to eat? Know that you can only sprint for 12 to 16 hours at a time, not for days. You also have plenty of time to eat a tasty and nutritious meal. Of course, some older women may need to eat regularly because of metabolic disorders or instructions on medications. In any case, you can speak to your doctor about your eating habits before making any adjustments.

Although it isn't actually fasting, some doctors say that allowing easy-to-digest foods like whole fruit during the fasting window has health benefits. Modifications like these will also provide a much-needed break for your digestive and metabolic systems. For example, the famous weight-loss book "Fit for Life" recommended consuming only fruit after supper and before lunch.

In fact, according to the writers of this book, they had patients who only changed their eating habits by fasting for 12 to 16 hours per day. Despite not adhering to the diet's other guidelines or counting calories, they lost weight and improved their health. This plan may have succeeded precisely because dieters substituted junk food for whole foods. In either case, participants considered this dietary adjustment to be successful and simple to enforce. Traditionalists won't call this fasting, but it's good to realize that you have choices if you can't go without food for more than a few hours.

Intermittent Fasting Typical Findings

In the medical literature, Dr. Becky, a chiropractor, and over-50 wellness coach, says it's difficult to find any disadvantages to IF. She clarified that the blood sugar and insulin levels would drop to dangerously low levels during the fasting phase. Your body will rely on stored fat for energy if insulin's hormonal fat-storing signal is not present.

The National Library of Medicine has also released an analysis of women's health-related sporadic fast outcomes. Studies on the use of fasting as a method to minimize the risk of cancer, diabetes, and other metabolic disorders, as well as heart disease, are among the report's highlights.

Is Intermittent Fasting (IF) Your Best Fat-Loss Tool?

In any case, IF seems to function largely because it is relatively simple to obey. They say it helps them instinctively reduce calories and make healthier food decisions by reducing eating windows. According to some research, IF tends to encourage fat loss while sparing lean muscle mass, making it a better choice than simply reducing calories, carbs, or fat.

Of course, the majority of people combine IF with another weight-loss strategy. To lose weight, you might decide to eat 1,200 calories per day. It could be better to spread out 1,200 calories over two meals and two snacks rather than three meals and three snacks. If you've had difficulty losing weight because your diet didn't work or was too difficult to adhere to, you may want to try intermittent fasting.

Is Intermittent Fasting Healthy for Diabetics?

Do you want to try intermittent fasting to help you control your diabetes? Intermittent fasting is beginning to feel like the cure-all for just about every ailment, from weight loss to cardiovascular disease and even cancer. As a registered dietitian, I'm still wary of new eating trends because the majority of them lack scientific evidence. Even though research on intermittent fasting is rapidly expanding, there is still much to learn about this popular "diet."

Intermittent fasting has gotten a lot of attention lately because of its potential for preventing and treating type 2 diabetes.

More than 34 million people in the United States alone have diabetes, and the number is steadily increasing every year. Adopting a healthy diet, exercising regularly, and managing stress are all important aspects of diabetes management, but it's not always clear whether certain eating patterns are more beneficial than others.

Let's begin with the fundamentals of intermittent fasting. Most people think of intermittent fasting as a diet, but it's really more of an umbrella word for a range of eating habits that include some sort of fasting for a fixed period of time (for more on intermittent fasting, click here).

The regular time-restricted feeding method, in which people or mice are fed meals within a designated time frame during the day, typically an 8-hour feeding window and a 16-hour fasting window, is the subject of a lot of IF studies. For example, one might fast for 16 hours and then eat between 11 a.m. and 7 p.m.

The alternate-day fasting approach and the 5:2 fasting approach are two other common IF protocols. For ADF, you consume about 500 to 700 calories every other day, and eat a daily diet on non-fasting days. Fasting is limited to twice a week instead of every other day in the 5:2 method, which has a similar definition.

IF, regardless of method, can be a more appealing alternative to conventional methods of calorie reduction (e.g., counting calories or removing entire food groups) because it is less inconvenient, more versatile, and intuitive, particularly for people who miss breakfast or eat less on weekends.

When you fast, what happens to your body?

Intermittent fasting allows the body to engage in a mechanism known as metabolic switching. When a person fasts for 8 to 12 hours, metabolic switching takes place. The body runs out of glucose (also known as blood sugar) during this process and turns to burn ketone bodies for food, which it obtains by breaking down stored fat. Reduced inflammation, improved glucose regulation, and more adaptive stress response are some of the additional benefits of switching from glucose to ketones as a fuel source.

The metabolic changes that occur during fasting may give IF an advantage over other diets for weight loss and managing metabolic conditions like diabetes, according to researchers.

What are the advantages of intermittent fasting for diabetes?

Fasting has been shown to have a substantial effect on blood sugar levels, but what does the evidence say about intermittent fasting and diabetes in particular?

Let's start at the beginning...

What is the cause of diabetes?

Diabetes is a metabolic disorder in which people have difficulty absorbing or metabolizing carbohydrates. When we ingest carbohydrates, they are broken down into a simple sugar called glucose, which is then released into our bloodstream (also known as blood sugar) for our cells to use as fuel.

When glucose reaches our bloodstream, our bodies release insulin, which aids our muscles, liver, fat tissues, and brain in consuming glucose from the bloodstream and transferring it to our cells, where it can be burned for energy.

Obesity and excess weight gain, for example, can inhibit our cells' ability to use insulin, causing glucose to build up in the bloodstream and resulting in high blood sugar. Insulin resistance, the driving force behind prediabetes and type 2 diabetes, is the consequence of this disease.

Is intermittent fasting beneficial for diabetics?

The response isn't completely straightforward, as it is with a lot of nutrition-related issues. Currently, the bulk of IF and diabetes testing is performed on animals. Although this has provided some insight into how intermittent fasting may aid in the treatment of diabetes, human research is mixed.

In mice, IF increases insulin sensitivity and avoids obesity, according to animal studies. In humans, IF successfully treated insulin resistance and decreased hemoglobin A1C (a measure of blood sugar regulation for many months) in participants with insulin-dependent type 2 diabetes, according to a recent case report published in BMJ. Another positive outcome: after observing IF for several months, all of the participants in the study were able to discontinue their insulin medication completely.

In a recent clinical trial, men with prediabetes were randomly assigned to one of two groups: one followed a 6-hour timed feeding IF protocol for 5 weeks, while the other followed a 12-hour feeding protocol (a 12-hour window is typical eating for most people, think 8 a.m. to 8 p.m.). The men in the IF group had less insulin resistance than those in the 12-hour feeding group, according to the study's results. Regardless of the amount of weight lost during the study, the IF group had better results. In a related study involving 107 overweight and obese women, IF was found to boost glucose regulation.

However, according to a systematic analysis of existing research on IF and diabetes, multiple studies have shown that IF has no additional benefit for insulin resistance and hemoglobin A1C as compared to a conventional calorie-controlled diet.

It's worth mentioning that much of the research on IF has been conducted on overweight and obese people with insulin resistance, so the findings do not extend to people with diabetes who aren't obese. In addition, some studies have shown that IF is more advantageous to men than it is to women.

Basically, there aren't enough high-quality studies in diverse groups of men and women to claim definitively that IF is better for diabetes control than a conventional balanced diet. Furthermore, the optimal length, frequency, and intensity of fasting necessary to generate metabolic benefits that are particularly beneficial for people with diabetes have yet to be determined.

Finally, for people with diabetes, intermittent fasting can have some theoretical and research-backed disadvantages. So far, here's what we learned.

What are the drawbacks of intermittent fasting when it comes to diabetes?

Intermittent fasting has been found by many physicians, including myself, to intensify disordered eating behaviors in vulnerable people. Waiting too long to eat can cause changes in hunger hormones, as well as an increase in appetite and cravings. This can lead to overeating and, in some situations, binge eating in many people.

In terms of study, some studies have discovered that IF may increase binge eating in bulimic people. Others have discovered that IF can actually assist in the reduction of disordered eating in overweight and obese people.

As a result, the available evidence indicates that IF can be dangerous to people of average weight as well as those who have either undergone disordered eating habits or have been diagnosed with eating disorders. Women may also be more vulnerable to the harmful effects of intermittent fasting.

Long-term intermittent fasting in overweight and obese women resulted in a longer menstrual cycle and altered reproductive hormone levels in normal-weight women, according to a few reports. More study is required to fully understand the effect of IF on women's menstrual cycles, but this is something to bear in mind if you're thinking about giving it a try.

In addition, one study looked at how three weeks of IF affected overweight men and women. Men had greater glucose control than women, according to the results, but women had poorer glucose control.

Another point to bear in mind is that the majority of human research on intermittent fasting suggests balanced eating (rather than feasting) on non-restricted days. Even if you're losing weight, evidence suggests that overindulging on days when you're not fasting can be harmful to your wellbeing.

Intermittent fasting has also been linked to the following harmful side effects:

- constipation
- water retention
- dizziness
- general weakness
- increased feelings of hunger
- worse mood
- heightened irritability
- difficulties concentrating
- increased fatigue
- eating-related thoughts
- fear of loss of control and overeating during non-restricted days

Overall, more research is needed to fully understand the benefits and risks of intermittent fasting for people with diabetes, but some women, people with eating disorders, and people with a "normal" bodyweight might not be the best candidates for intermittent fasting. Before making substantial dietary changes, consult your health care team or a registered dietitian for more detailed advice.

Intermittent Fasting and Your Menstrual Cycle.

Women who fast on a regular basis may be concerned about how fasting affects their menstrual cycle, hormones, and reproductive health as intermittent fasting becomes more common. Although there is little research on how intermittent fasting or ketogenic diets influence human reproductive cycles, research on other metabolic and lifestyle characteristics and behaviors such as weight, exercise, and caloric restriction can provide some insight.

Caloric restriction, for example, is a "stressor" that is stored in the brain and can affect sex hormone release via the hypothalamic-pituitary-gonadal (HPG) axis. Hormones in the HPG axis regulate reproduction and fertility.

When it comes to intermittent fasting, it's likely that people who don't eat enough calories to sustain the hypothalamic-pituitary-gonadal axis will have irregular menses.

This means that if a woman doesn't have enough nutritional or metabolic resources to bear a baby, her body can send a warning to her brain to turn off the reproductive cycle. As a result, women who are attempting to conceive should avoid fasting for more than 24 hours at a time or restricting their caloric intake substantially through fasting, especially if they are already at a healthy weight / BMI. A few days of fasting each month is unlikely to interrupt your menstrual cycle, however extreme caloric restriction may.

Negative energy balance or caloric restriction in very young women can also have an effect on the HPG axis and neurohormones, delaying puberty.

We all know that losing weight and even exercising too often will result in irregular or absent menstrual cycles.

From the moment we get our first period until we hit menopause, our reproductive systems are capable of sustaining a pregnancy. In order to sustain a healthy pregnancy, women need a certain amount of energy and nutrients, which must be derived from food and preserved as fat. When these energy stores are exhausted, our bodies have the ability to sense this and, in effect, 'turn off' our reproductive cycles, preventing pregnancy. The mechanism is actually very complicated, and it necessitates a delicate balance of signals being exchanged between the brain, pituitary gland, and ovaries. Normal menstrual cycles typically return after a woman regains weight and/or resumes a nutrient-rich diet.

How long will I go without eating without impacting my period?

It would be difficult to come up with any general rules for how many days of fasting a month, for example, would be healthy for a woman seeking to conceive or to stop any menstrual cycle adjustments. For instance, menstrual cycles differ significantly from person to person. Although moderate time-restricted feeding (around 12-14 hours a day or less) or occasional fasting periods under 24 hours are probably healthy, the effects of intermittent fasting and ketogenic diets on reproductive health are likely to be determined by diet consistency, caloric intake, and BMI.

"If your intermittent fasting causes food shortages or long-term low blood sugar or hypoglycemia, it will most likely affect the hypothalamic-pituitary–gonadal axis, disrupting reproductive hormone output.

Chapter 3: Types of IF

Fasting isn't just a scientifically established form of weight reduction. Fasting diets of different forms assist in the elimination of cellular waste and can also boost your mood. You may benefit from fasting in several ways, from lowering your risk of disease to improving your memory.

Fasting can be integrated into any diet, but if you need structure, there are many choices. You'll find a style that works for you based on your eating patterns and fitness goals. Continue reading to discover some of the most successful fasting diets and how to get started.

WHAT ARE FASTING DIETARY REQUIREMENTS?

Fasting diets usually include a period of fasting (abstaining from eating or drinking something with calories) and a period of eating, often based on particular food classes, though there is no one-size-fits-all solution.

You could miss breakfast a few days a week or limit your eating window every day if you're on this diet. It's completely up to you to find out what works best for you.

Fasting diets affect everyone differently, but this way of eating can make you feel more like yourself. Fasting diets can help you control your weight and boost your mood. Other advantages include better memory and alertness, as well as autophagy, the body's natural way of eliminating damaged cells and toxins to make room for new, healthier cells.

FASTING DIETS RULES

During your eating window, cutting back on carbohydrates and filling up on the right fats will help you prevent blood sugar crashes that occur during fasting times. Try a range of fasting diet foods and see how you do.

Drink plenty of water to keep hydrated. Make an attempt to absorb more water than normal.

If you want to exercise, plan your meals to correspond with your workout. Some people tend to go to the gym instead of eating while they're fasting. Do what you think is best for you.

If you're going to break your fast, make it a good one. To optimize your nutrient intake, the best fasting diet foods are balanced whole foods like fruits, quality fats, and pasture-raised meat.

To help you get through your quick, stock up on your favorite beverages. On fasting days, you can drink plain tea and coffee, such as clean Bulletproof Coffee Beans, unless you're doing a strict water-only fast.

When the energy levels dip on non-fasting days, have high-fat, lower-carb snacks and beverages on hand, such as a Bulletproof Collagen Protein Bar or a Bulletproof Cold Brew Latte.

TYPES OF INTERMITTENT FASTING

16:8 FASTING DIET
This is an intermittent fasting diet in which you eat only for eight hours a day, generally between noon and eight p.m.

- Limit carbs to dinner and drink plenty of water during the day for best performance.
- To get even more intermittent fasting advantages, try an 18-hour fast with a six-hour eating window after you've gotten used to a 16-hour fast.

One of the most common fasting diets is the 16:8 diet. It's a fantastic way to ease into fasting for those who are new to it. During your eating window, Simple 16:8 does not limit your food choices. A lower-carb diet rich in nutrient-dense foods, on the other hand, will help you produce better results.

Since a low-carb diet keeps your blood sugar levels steady, it's easier to stop feeling "angry" during your fast, which is one of the most common negative side effects of fasting. A lower-carb diet also makes it easier to enter ketosis, which has the added advantage of reducing hunger.

5:2 FASTING DIET
- Five days a week, eat normally. Limit calories to 500-600 per day on two days per week.
- On calorie-restricted days, eat three small meals or two slightly larger meals.
- Fasting days can be spread out between eating days to help you feel less hungry.

When opposed to calorie restriction alone, studies show that 5:2 fasting can lead to weight loss and increased insulin tolerance (which can lower the risk of type 2 diabetes).

STOP EATING FASTING DIET
- Twice a week, fast for 24 hours and eat normally the other five days.
- Consume healthy foods on daily eating days.
- You will continue to eat every day. On Friday, eat at 7 a.m., start your fast at 8 a.m., and eat again after 8:00 a.m.

The Eat Stop Eat fasting diet, according to author Brad Pilon's experience, helps you to eat normally for the majority of the week. Fasting for 24 hours twice a week will help kickstart ketosis by generating a calorie deficit. A 24-hour fast, on the other hand, is a long period of time, and you should consult your doctor before attempting longer fasts.

4:3 FASTING DIET (AKA ALTERNATE DAY FASTING)
- Fast every other day and eat normally on the days when you aren't fasting. You'll eat normally for four days and fast for three, or vice versa, over the course of a week.
- Limit yourself to 500 calories on fasting days.

- On non-fasting days, eat normally.

The 4:3 diet could help you lose weight. However, with too much fasting, sticking to the diet can be challenging. According to a study, this fasting diet induces hunger and irritability, which may prevent you from sticking to it long-term. On fasting days, keep busy and distracted to stay on track.

- WARRIOR DIET
- For a 20-hour period, fast or eat less than you usually do, then eat one big meal during a four-hour evening window.
- You can consume small quantities of raw produce like berries or leafy greens, zero-calorie drinks like green tea, or protein-like poached eggs during the fasting time.
- Eat wholesome, organic, high-nutrient foods for your evening meal.

The Warrior Diet is based on author Ori Hofmekler's experiences in the Israeli Special Forces as well as his observations regarding ancient warriors' dietary habits, rather than hard science. Depending on how much you limit your food consumption and what you consume during the eating window, the Warrior Diet results can differ drastically.

- ONE MEAL A DAY (OMAD)
- Eat your daily calories in a one-hour window after fasting for 23 hours.
- Try eating between 4 and 7 p.m. every day to provide ample time to socialize while still digesting before bedtime.
- When you do eat, make sure it's a safe, balanced meal rather than a giant pizza.

OMAD helps you to reap all of the benefits of fasting while still simplifying your routine and eating habits. Since OMAD requires calorie restriction and only eating one meal a day, it will help you get the most out of a fasting diet. Since OMAD takes more time, wait until you've had more fasting experience before attempting it.

- SPONTANEOUS MEAL SKIPPING

When you aren't hungry, miss meals.

When you do eat, adhere to your daily eating routine.

This fasting diet takes an intuitive approach, making it suitable for those looking for maximum versatility. During non-fasting hours, eat a diet low in carbohydrates and high in quality fats, such as the keto diet, to maintain a healthy weight, keep your blood sugar stable, and even prolong your fasting window.

Chapter 4: Food to Eat and To Avoid

INTERMITTENT FASTING entails switching between eating and fasting periods.

Intermittent fasting, according to advocates, is a healthy and effective way to lose weight and boost your health."

Intermittent fasting is a term that refers to an eating pattern that alternates between periods of fasting and non-fasting for a fixed period of time.

Time-restricted eating is one of the most common methods. It advises eating only for eight hours a day and fasting for the remaining 16 hours. It can help us lose weight while also allowing our gut and hormones to rest in between meals during our fast.

The 5:2 method, in which you eat normally and healthily for five days a week, is another common strategy. You only eat one meal a day for the other two days of the week, which should be between 500 and 700 calories." This helps our bodies to relax while also reducing the amount of calories we eat during the week.

Intermittent fasting has been related to weight loss, increased cholesterol, blood sugar regulation, and reduced inflammation in research.

According to a study published in the New England Journal of Medicine in 2019, "preclinical and clinical studies have shown that intermittent fasting has broad-spectrum benefits for many health problems, such as obesity, (diabetes), cardiovascular disease, cancers, and neurologic disorders." According to the report, clinical research has mainly concentrated on overweight young and middle-aged adults.

It's crucial to apply the same fundamental nutrition principles to intermittent fasting as to other healthy eating plans." In 120 nations, the organization offers nutrition education and resources to health and wellness practitioners as well as individual customers.

"In fact, these (principles) might be even more relevant when you're going without food for longer periods of time, which can lead to overeating in some people.

If you're on an intermittent fasting schedule, here are some instructions to follow:

- Most of the time, eat minimally processed foods.
- Consume a range of foods, including lean protein, vegetables, fruits, smart carbs, and healthy fats.
- Make flavorful, delicious meals for yourself.

Slowly and mindfully eat your meals until you're happy.

Diets based on intermittent fasting do not require complex menus. However, adhering to healthy eating standards, there are some items that should be eaten and those that should be avoided.

On an intermittent fasting diet, you can eat the following three foods:

- Lean proteins.
- Fruits.
- Vegetables.

Lean Proteins

Eating lean protein keeps you fuller for longer than other foods and lets you sustain or grow muscle.

Here are five protein sources that are both lean and healthy:

- Chicken breast.
- Plain Greek yogurt.
- Beans, peas, and lentils.
- Fish and shellfish.
- Tofu and tempeh.

Fruits

Intermittent fasting, like every other eating schedule, necessitates the intake of high-nutrient foods. Vitamins, minerals, phytonutrients (plant nutrients), and fiber are commonly found in fruits and vegetables. These vitamins, minerals, and nutrients can assist in the reduction of cholesterol, blood sugar regulation, and bowel health. Another advantage is the low-calorie content of fruits and vegetables.

According to the government's 2015-20 Dietary Recommendations for Americans, most people should consume about 2 cups of fruit a day on a 2,000-calorie diet.

Here are ten good fruits to eat while fasting intermittently:

- Apples.
- Apricots.
- Blueberries.
- Blackberries.
- Cherries.
- Peaches.
- Pears.
- Plums.
- Oranges.
- Watermelon.
- Vegetables

Vegetables will help you adhere to your intermittent fasting schedule. A diet high in leafy greens has been shown to lower the risk of heart disease, Type 2 diabetes, cancer, cognitive decline, and other diseases. According to the government's 2015-20 Dietary Recommendations for Americans, most people can consume 2.5 cups of vegetables a day on a 2,000-calorie diet.

Here are six vegetables that would be helpful to include in a balanced intermittent eating plan:

- Kale.
- Spinach.
- Chard.
- Cabbage.
- Collard greens.
- Arugula.

Foods to avoid

Certain foods should not be eaten as part of an intermittent fasting procedure. You can avoid foods that are high in sugar, fat, and salt since they are high in calories. They won't satisfy you after a short, and they might even make you hungry. They also have very little nutrition.

Avoid the following foods if you want to adhere to an intermittent eating plan:

- Snack chips.
- Microwave popcorn.

Foods with a lot of added sugar can also be avoided. Sugar in processed foods and beverages is devoid of nutrients and amounts to sweet, empty calories, which is not what you want if you're fasting intermittently. Sugar metabolizes very rapidly, so it will make you hungry.

If you're doing intermittent fasting, stay away from sugary foods like:

- Cookies.
- Candy.
- Cakes.
- Barbecue sauce and ketchup.
- Fruit juice.
- Sugary cereals and granola.

Chapter 5: Super Foods to Eat for Woman Over 50

Foods with a high nutrient value are known as superfoods. This means they provide a lot of nutrients for a limited amount of calories.

Minerals, vitamins, and antioxidants are abundant in them.

Antioxidants are natural molecules present in a number of foods. They aid in the neutralization of free radicals in our bodies. Free radicals are natural byproducts of energy production that can cause severe health problems.

The goal of maintaining an optimally balanced and active mind and body in youth is to prevent disease by maintaining a body that can procreate.

To be in the best possible shape, we must pay attention to what we eat as we get older. "As we age, our metabolism slows, and our bodies' ability to break down and use their fuel sources declines.

Furthermore, some vitamins are becoming increasingly essential in helping to protect against diseases and health problems.

Here are some foods to consume to keep the body and mind in good condition.

1. Foods high in fiber, such as raspberries

Unfortunately, this is something you might already be aware of: when you grow older, your gastrointestinal function slows down, so it's important to concentrate on eating enough fiber to keep your system going.

Fiber not only increases gastrointestinal efficiency, but it also reduces gastrointestinal inflammation and cholesterol thus offering a gradual release of energy-rich carbohydrates into the bloodstream. Older women and men can strive for 25 to 30 grams of fiber per day.

The Mayo Clinic recommends raspberries, which have 8 grams of fiber per cup; whole wheat pasta, which has 6.3 grams per cup; lentils, which have 15.6 grams per cup; and green peas, which have 8.8 grams per cup.

2. Corn flakes and other foods rich in B12

Stomach acid helps release vitamin B12 from food, and B12 is vital because it helps maintain a healthy nervous system and key metabolic processes. As we age, our stomach acidity decreases, making it more difficult to get enough vitamin B12 in our diet.

10 to 30% of adults over the age of 50 have trouble consuming vitamin B12 from food." "People who take antacids or other drugs that inhibit stomach acid may have trouble absorbing vitamin B12 from food." People over 50 should get 2.4 micrograms of B12 every day.

Animal-derived foods, such as beef, eggs, fish, and dairy, produce the most B12, but B12-fortified foods, such as whole-grain cereals, also contain the vitamin. Consult your doctor about adding a multivitamin or B12 supplement to your diet if you're concerned about not having enough B12.

3. Cinnamon and turmeric

Another thing that disappears as we age is our sense of taste. "Because saliva development and taste sensitivity decrease with age, you may want to start experimenting with different spices, like turmeric."

"Turmeric has been shown to increase immune function, minimize joint inflammation, and prevent arthritis in elderly people. Turmeric, and its main active compound curcumin, has been shown in other studies to have a real impact on preventing Alzheimer's disease and certain cancers.

Cinnamon is another spice to add to your spice cabinet. "Cinnamon is well-known for its anti-inflammatory and antibacterial properties.

Cinnamon also aids blood sugar regulation by slowing the rate at which the stomach empties after meals, thus balancing blood sugar highs and lows. Studies also indicate that cinnamon can be used therapeutically for type 2 diabetes, as it tends to enhance the body's insulin sensitivity.

4. Drinking water

As we age, our sense of taste diminishes, as does our thirst, making dehydration more normal.

Women should drink nine cups of water a day, while men should drink 13 cups," says the National Institutes of Health. You'll need more if you're more physically involved and live in a hotter environment.

5. potassium-rich foods include bananas and other potassium-rich foods.

It's a fact that as we grow older, our risk of stroke and heart disease rises. Eat foods rich in potassium, such as bananas and avocados, to help lower your risk.

A new analysis of women aged 50 to 70 showed that those who ingested the most potassium had the lowest chance of experiencing a stroke. According to the World Health Organization, potassium will also help to reduce blood pressure.

The minimum daily potassium intake is 4,700 milligrams. Potassium-rich foods include potatoes, which contain approximately 900 milligrams per potato; bananas, which contain 400 milligrams per banana; avocado, which contains over 700 milligrams per cup; and pistachios, which contain 1,200 milligrams per cup.

6. Foods high in calcium

Calcium is best known for its role in the formation and maintenance of strong bones and teeth, but it is also necessary for proper heart, muscle, and nervous system function.

The goal for men and women is to consume 1,200 milligrams per day, but intake is a challenge for both men and women due to two factors:

Lactose sensitivity, which is normal as people age, can make having enough calcium a challenge.

"Research has shown that as you age, your access to sunlight as well as vitamin D-rich foods, combined with consuming D less effectively, both lead to slightly below-normal levels of this all-important vitamin.

If you're lactose intolerant, eat leafy greens like collards, mustard, kale, and bok choy. "You can also try canned salmon (with bones) and sardines, as well as tofu made with a calcium compound," says the source.

Request a vitamin D test from your doctor to ensure you are getting enough vitamin D. The target range is 50-70 nmol/L. If your D level is poor, you can improve it by consuming D-rich foods, having 15 minutes of sun per day, and taking a supplement prescribed by your doctor.

7. Broccoli and other leafy greens are good sources of iron.

As you get older, it's more important to protect your eyes, particularly because many eye problems come with it. Lutein, which is linked to beta carotene and vitamin A, is a vital nutrient for healthy vision and the prevention of macular degeneration. And most people over the age of 50 can't seem to get enough of it. Lutein is found in green leafy plants, as well as apples, bananas, and egg yolks.

Some Food Ideas

Apart from incorporating the foods mentioned above in your diet, It is recommended that adopting these general healthy-eating guidelines:

Focus on healthy fats derived from nuts, lean meats, fish, low-fat dairy, olive oil, and plant-based sources like avocados to reduce saturated fats and prevent cardiovascular disease.

Since your metabolism slows when you grow older, you'll need to change how many calories you consume on a regular basis. Even if you're a busy guy, you should do this. The general range is 1,400-2,400 calories a day, with men eating more calories.

Cookies, chips, candies, cookies, and pastries are examples of refined, processed foods and beverages that should be avoided or reduced. These refined foods increase inflammation in the body, increasing the risk of cancer, diabetes, and heart disease.

Supplements and a multivitamin are two choices. Supplements are relevant for seniors in general, but you can speak to your doctor about what you're taking. A gender- and an age-specific multivitamin is also required in addition to the supplements.

Chapter 6: Mistakes to avoid during IF

1. GETTING STARTED QUICKLY WITH INTERMITTENT FASTING

One of the biggest mistakes you can make is to start off too fast. You will set yourself up for failure if you jump into IF without first easing into it. It can be difficult to switch from consuming three big meals or six small meals a day to eating within a four-hour window, for example.

Instead, gradually introduce fasting. If you choose to use the 16/8 process, progressively increase the time between meals until you can work comfortably in a 12-hour window. Then, to get the window down to 8 hours, add a few minutes per day before you get there.

2. CHOOSING THE WRONG INTERMITTENT FASTING PLAN

You've shopped for whole foods like fish and poultry, fruits and vegetables, and nutritious sides like quinoa and legumes, and you're eager to try Intermittent Fasting for weight loss. The issue is that you haven't selected the IF approach that will ensure your success. If you go to the gym six days a week, absolutely fasting for two of those days might not be the best idea for you.

Rather than rushing into a plan without thinking about it, assess your lifestyle and select the plan that best fits your schedule and behaviors.

3. EXCESSIVE EATING IN YOUR FASTING WINDOW

The decreased time available to eat means eating less calories, which is one of the reasons people want to pursue Intermittent Fasting. Some people, on the other hand, will eat their normal amount of calories during the fasting window. It's likely that you won't lose weight as a result of this.

Don't eat your normal calorie intake of 2000 calories in the slot. Instead, strive for a caloric intake of 1200 to 1500 calories during the time you're breaking the quick. If you fast for 4, 6, or 8 hours, the amount of meals you consume will be determined by the duration of the fasting window. If you find yourself in a state of starvation and need to feed, rethink the diet you want to pursue, or take a day off the IF to refocus and then get back on track.

4. EATING THE WRONG FOODS IN YOUR FASTING WINDOW

Overeating goes hand in hand with the Intermittent Fasting error of eating the wrong foods. You would not feel good if you have a fasting window of 6 hours and fill it with processed, fatty, or sugary foods.

The mainstay of your diet becomes lean proteins, healthy fats, nuts, legumes, unrefined grains, and wholesome vegetables and fruits. In addition, when you're not fasting, keep these safe eating tips in mind:

- Rather than dining at a restaurant, cook and eat at home.

- Read nutrition labels to learn about ingredients like high fructose corn syrup and refined palm oil that aren't authorized.
- Keep an eye out for secret sugars and limit your sodium intake.
- Instead of processed foods, prepare whole foods.
- Fiber, balanced carbs and fats, and lean proteins should all be present on your plate.

5. CALORIE RESTRICTION IN YOUR FASTING WINDOW

Yeah, there is such a thing as calorie restriction that is unnecessary. It's not safe to eat less than 1200 calories during your fasting window. Not only that, but it has the ability to slow down your metabolic rate. If you slow your metabolism too much, you'll start losing muscle mass instead of adding it.

To avoid making this error, prepare your meals for the week ahead on the weekend. You'll have balanced, nutritious meals at your fingertips in no time. When it's time to eat, you can choose from a range of good, nutritious, and calorie-balanced options.

6. BREAKING THE INTERMITTENT FAST WITHOUT REALIZING IT

It's important to be aware of secret fast breakers. Did you know that even the taste of sugar makes the brain release insulin? This triggers the release of insulin, effectively breaking the fast. Here are some unexpected foods, supplements, and products that can stop a fast and activate an insulin response:

- Supplements containing maltodextrin and pectin as well as other additives
- Sugar and fat are present in vitamins such as gummy bear vitamins.
- Using toothpaste and mouthwash with xylitol as a sweetener
- Sugar can be present in the coating of pain relievers like Advil.
- Breaking your fast is a common Intermittent Fasting error. When you're not eating, brush your teeth with a baking soda and water paste, and read the labels carefully before taking vitamins and supplements.

7. DRINKING INSUFFICIENTLY DURING INTERMITTENT FASTING

IF necessitates that you remain hydrated. Bear in mind that your body isn't consuming the water that would usually be absorbed with food. As a consequence, if you're not careful, side effects can throw you off. If you allow yourself to become dehydrated, you can experience headaches, muscle cramps, and extreme hunger.

Include the following in your day to prevent this error and avoid painful symptoms like cramping and headaches:

- Water
- 2 Tbsp Apple Cider Vinegar and Water (This May Even Curb Your Hunger)
- A Cup of Black Coffee
- Green Tea, Black Tea, Herbal Tea, Oolong

8. WHEN INTERMITTENTLY FASTING, DO NOT EXERCISE.

Some people assume they can't exercise during an IF time, when in fact, it's the ideal situation. Exercising helps you burn fat that has been accumulated in your body. Additionally, when you exercise, the Human Growth Hormone levels rise, assisting in muscle growth. There are, however, certain rules to obey in order to get the best out of your workouts.

Keep the following points in mind to get the best results from your efforts:

Time your workouts to coincide with meal times, and then eat healthy carbohydrates and proteins within 30 minutes of completing your workout.

If the workout is strenuous, make sure you eat beforehand to replenish your glycogen reserves.

Focus your workout on your fasting method; if you're fasting for 24 hours, don't do something strenuous that day. Keep hydrated during the fast and particularly during the workout.

Pay attention to your body's signals; if you start to feel weak or light-headed, take a rest or stop working out.

9. BEING TOO HARD ON YOURSELF IF YOU SLIP WHEN INTERMITTENT FASTING

One blunder does not equal disaster! You'll have days when an IF diet is particularly difficult and you don't think you'll be able to keep up. It's perfectly appropriate to take a break if necessary. Set aside a day to refocus. Stick to the balanced eating schedule, but indulge in treats like an amazing protein smoothie or a helping of healthy beef and broccoli the next day.

Don't fall into the pit of allowing Intermittent Fasting to take over your whole life. Consider it a part of your good lifestyle, and don't forget to take care of yourself in other ways. Enjoy a good read, get some exercise, spend quality time with your family, and eat as healthily as possible. It's just part of the process of being the best version of yourself.

Chapter 7: Autophagy of IF

Fasting, which entails reducing calorie consumption for an extended period of time, tends to have some pretty impressive health benefits. Weight loss, increases in diabetes and heart disease risk factors, and a longer life span are among them.

For years, scientists have been trying to find out why fasting is related to longevity. Fasting lab mice and monkeys have a propensity to live longer than their regularly fed counterparts.

According to a study, calorie restriction stimulates genes that tell cells to recycle energy. The cells enter a preservation or "famine" phase, which makes them surprisingly immune to disease and cellular stress. They also begin autophagy, a process in which the body cleans out old, discarded, and unneeded cellular material while also restoring and recycling damaged parts.

In one study, mice that went without food for 24 hours had a lot of autophagosomes, which suggests autophagy is working. Since mouse metabolism is much faster than ours, we must be wary about applying this directly to humans. While autophagy is difficult to assess outside of a lab setting, many experts agree that the autophagy process in humans starts after 18-20 hours of fasting, with the greatest benefits occurring after 48–72 hours. If this sounds overwhelming, bear in mind that intermittent fasting will still offer benefits, but you may want to consider a longer fast once in a while (a few times a year depending on your specific risk factors) to completely trigger autophagy and do some spring cleaning for your cells. Of course, before starting any fasting regimen, you should always check with your doctor.

Autophagy stimulation accomplishes two goals: it cleans out old, unwanted cellular materials and proteins and it stimulates the development of growth hormone, which regenerates new cellular material and fuels cell regeneration. Autophagy may be able to kill remaining bacteria or viruses if the body has recently been contaminated.

Not only has autophagy been related to improved survival, but it is also assisting researchers in better understanding degenerative disorders like Parkinson's and Alzheimer's. When autophagy is infrequent, the body accumulates a variety of cellular material, including proteins such as amyloid-beta or Tau protein, which are present in large amounts in Alzheimer's, Parkinson's, and even cancer. Long bouts of autophagy, according to researchers, could be able to rid the brain of excess proteins, possibly preventing the development of diseases like Alzheimer's and Parkinson's.

What is the safest way to accomplish autophagy?

While some diet and fitness blogs believe that some supplements can induce autophagy, there is only one known way to activate it: fasting. Autophagy is caused by nutrient deprivation.

When the body's nutrients are exhausted, autophagy signaling includes two main pathways:

The nutrients that affect cellular development, protein synthesis, and anabolism are regulated by mTOR or mammalian target of rapamycin. It has been related to the activation of insulin receptors and the development of new tissue.

AMPK, or AMP-activated protein kinase, is a protein that helps the body maintain energy homeostasis and activate its backup fuel systems.

Both mTOR and AMPK are sensitive to nutrient levels in the body. These two pathways determine whether your body will activate a growth response (mTor) or enter autophagy (AMPK).

Autophagy also cooperates with two essential hormones: glucagon and insulin. People with diabetes or hypoglycemia have difficulty managing their blood sugar levels or are overly sensitive to insulin. Insulin causes glucagon to decrease, and vice versa. When you fast, your insulin levels drop and your glucagon levels rise, stimulating autophagy.

However, it's not quite that simple: low liver glycogen is needed to induce autophagy, which is normally only done after 14–16 hours of fasting but is even more likely after 24 hours, so it's a major commitment.

Despite these wonderful advantages, the degree of fasting needed to enable autophagy is not suitable for everyone. During such fasts, some people feel tired, irritable, and have trouble sleeping. Do check in with your healthcare providers and aim for balance.

All You Need to Know About Autophagy

Autophagy is a crucial process in which the cells of the body "clean out" any unwanted or damaged materials.

Autophagy has been related to a variety of health benefits by researchers. Fasting may also be able to cause autophagy, according to the researchers.

It's important to bear in mind, however, that much of the autophagy research is still in its early stages.

There are trillions of cells in a person's body. Unwanted molecules will accumulate within them over time, causing damage to some of their components.

Autophagy is a natural process that responds to this issue, according to a 2015 article published in Nature. The cells eliminate these unwanted molecules and defective sections during autophagy.

Any of these molecules and sections are often killed by autophagy. At other times, the cell recycles these components to produce new ones.

The expression "autophagy" comes from the Ancient Greek word "autophagy," which means "self-eating."

Impact on health

Autophagy has been related to a number of health benefits in research, but since this cellular mechanism is so complex, it can be difficult to draw conclusions.

A recent 2019 study, for example, surveyed current autophagy and cancer studies. Autophagy can help cancer cells stall their development, but it can also encourage their growth, depending on the stage of the tumor.

The relation between autophagy and liver health is also of interest to researchers. Autophagy can help protect liver cells from drug and alcohol-induced liver injury, according to a review article published in 2020.

According to other studies, autophagy is involved in a number of liver functions and can help to prevent the development of many liver diseases, including:

- Wilson's disease
- acute liver injury
- nonalcoholic fatty liver disease
- chronic alcohol-related liver disease

However, the bulk of autophagy research has been performed in test tubes or animal models. More research in humans is required, according to the authors of the study above, to determine how autophagy affects care.

Autophagy also appears to be critical in the immune system, as it eliminates toxins and infectious agents.

Autophagy has been shown to enhance the prognosis of cells with infectious and neurodegenerative diseases by reducing inflammation.

Autophagy assists in the defense of cells against incoming pathogens, according to another review report.

While there is a lot of research on autophagy's impact on cells, scientists aren't sure whether improving autophagy might be a new therapy for a number of diseases.

Fasting is linked

While autophagy occurs naturally in the body, many people wonder if it can be induced by the use of specific triggers.

Autophagy can be caused by fasting. If anyone fasts, they willingly go without food for a prolonged period of time — hours, days, or even weeks.

Orthodox calorie restriction is not the same as fasting. When anyone limits their calorie consumption, they are reducing their daily food intake. Depending on how much food a person eats during feeding times, fasting can or may not result in calorie restriction.

Fasting and calorie restriction can also cause autophagy, according to a 2018 review of the existing literature.

While some evidence of this process in humans exists, the majority of this research concentrates on non-human animals.

The cells of the body are stressed by fasting and calorie restriction. When anyone reduces the amount of food they eat, their cells receive less calories than they need to function properly.

As a consequence, the cells must become more effective. Autophagy allows the body's cells to scrub out and recycle any unused or damaged parts in response to the stress induced by fasting or calorie restriction.

However, scientists are unsure which cells respond in this way to fasting and calorie restriction. Those attempting to induce autophagy by fasting should be mindful that fat cells, for example, may not be targeted.

Fasting has yet to be shown to cause autophagy in the brain, according to researchers. Short-term fasting can cause autophagy in brain cells, according to at least one animal study.

Is it possible to cause autophagy?

Autophagy is caused by placing cells under tension, which is induced by fasting and calorie restriction. Researchers suspect, however, that there might be other ways to cause autophagy.

Exercising puts the body's cells under tension as well. The components of people's cells become weakened and inflamed when they exercise. Our cells react to this problem with autophagy, according to the authors of one study.

This indicates that people might be able to cause autophagy through exercise. Exercise does, in fact, tend to enhance autophagy in human skeletal muscles.

Curcumin intake has also been related to autophagy, at least in mouse studies, according to researchers. Curcumin is a naturally occurring chemical present in the turmeric root, a commonly used spice.

Curcumin-induced restoration of autophagy, for example, has been shown to protect against diabetic cardiomyopathy, a heart muscle disease that affects people with diabetes.

Curcumin was found to help mice battle cognitive dysfunction induced by chemotherapy by inducing autophagy in particular brain regions, according to another study.

While these preliminary results are encouraging, scientists must perform further study before drawing any conclusions. Scientists are unsure if increasing curcumin intake will cause autophagy in humans.

Chapter 8: Manage menopause

Here are five remedies for five symptoms that are common among women in their forties and fifties. (Remember, any questions you have should always be discussed with your healthcare provider first.) Other medications or potentially adverse side effects can be available. You should decide the choices are better for you as a couple.)

1. Mood Changes

Hormone fluctuations during perimenopause can leave some women feeling out of control. Increased irritability, anxiety, exhaustion, and depressed moods are common complaints. Relaxation and stress-reduction strategies, such as deep-breathing exercises and massage, as well as a healthy lifestyle (including good diet and physical exercise) and fun, self-nurturing activities, can all be beneficial. Some people use over-the-counter remedies like St. John's wort or vitamin B6 to alleviate menopause symptoms.

Discussing your mood problems with your doctor will help you figure out what's causing them, check for serious depression, and decide on the best course of action. Prescription antidepressant drugs can be prescribed for depression to remedy a chemical imbalance. While it takes many weeks to feel the full effect of one of these treatments, several women report significant improvements with very few side effects. Hot flashes have been shown to be treated by certain antidepressants. When antidepressant treatment is combined with counseling or psychotherapy, it is most effective.

2. Urinary Incontinence

Although urinary incontinence is described as the involuntary loss of urine over time, most women would describe it as an unfortunate, unexpected, and unwanted nuisance. Fortunately, there are non-surgical and non-medication methods for treating different types of incontinence. To keep urine filtered (clear and pale yellow), drink plenty of water and avoid foods or drinks rich in acid or caffeine, which can irritate the bladder lining. Grapefruit, bananas, tomatoes, coffee, and caffeine-containing soft drinks are among them. To strengthen the pelvic floor muscles and reduce incontinence episodes, try Kegel exercises.

3. Sweats at Night

Try these various ways to stay calm while sleeping to get relief from night sweats (hot flashes that occur during sleep):

- Dress in light nightclothes.
- Use layered bedding that can easily be removed during the night.
- Or, try wicking materials for both.
- Cool down with an electric fan.
- Sip cool water throughout the night

Keep a frozen cold pack under your pillow and flip it over often so your head is always resting on a cool surface, or place a cold pack on your feet.

4. Having a Hard Time Falling Asleep
Establish a consistent sleep schedule and routine:

- Even on weekends, get up and go to bed at the same times every day.
- Before going to bed, unwind and relax by reading a book, listening to music, or taking a long bath.
- Tryptophan is found in milk and peanuts, and it helps the body relax.
- A cup of chamomile tea could also help.
- Maintain a comfortable amount of light, noise, and temperature in your bedroom — dark, quiet, and cool are conducive to sleep.
- Use the bedroom for sleeping and sex.
- Avoid caffeine and alcohol.

5. Sexual Dissatisfaction
Menopause causes changes in sexual function by reducing ovarian hormone output, which can cause vaginal dryness and a decline in sexual function. To combat these changes, try the following:

Vaginal lubricants: These drugs, which are available without a prescription, reduce pressure and make intercourse easier when the vagina is dry. Since oil-based products like Vaseline can irritate the skin, only water-soluble products should be used. Just use vaginal products; avoid hand creams and lotions that contain alcohol or perfumes, as well as warming/tingling and flavored lubricants that may irritate sensitive tissue. (Astroglide, Moist Again, and Silk-E are some of the vaginal lubricants available.)

Vaginal moisturizers: These items, which are often available without a prescription, help people with moderate vaginal atrophy preserve or increase vaginal moisture (when tissues of the vulva and the lining of the vagina become thin, dry, less elastic, and less lubricated as a result of estrogen loss). They also keep the pH of the vaginal environment low, ensuring a safe vaginal environment. Replens and K-Y Long-lasting Vaginal Moisturizer are two examples.) These drugs are more long-lasting than vaginal lubricants and can be used on a regular basis.

Last but not least, women can maintain vaginal health by engaging in painless sexual activity on a regular basis, which increases blood flow to the genital region.

Menopause Natural Treatments That Actually Work

Women who don't want to use hormone therapy to relieve their menopause symptoms have a number of options that can be very successful. For memory issues, weight gain, high cholesterol, and vaginal symptoms, here are some natural lifestyle tips.

Natural Remedies: A Word of Caution

Always keep in mind that normally does not imply risk-free. Many herbal, fruit and dietary supplements may interfere with prescription drugs or worsen chronic medical conditions. Natural methods are not without risk, and the more you know, the better equipped you will be to select therapies that will keep you healthy and secure.

Check with your medical professional before choosing to use alternative and complementary treatments for your menopause symptoms, and read up on any potential side effects and cautions for any remedy you're considering.

Memory Problems

It's aggravating to try to remember a word or name that's on the tip of your tongue but you can't get it out. As you prepare to leave the house, forgetting where you put your car keys or where you put your glasses will drive you insane. Does this ring a bell? When they approach perimenopause, many women begin to notice memory problems. There are things you can do to keep your memory when you grow older, even though it's just the normal aging process.

Green tea consumption has been linked to a variety of health benefits, including the enhancement of the immune system and the prevention of cancer. Green tea is now being linked to preventing memory-damaging enzyme activity in studies. It has a small number of side effects and is widely available.

A sufficient amount of sleep is needed for your brain to process memory tasks. Both short and longer naps seem to help memory work, according to research. If you can't get a cat nap during the day, make sure you get enough overnight sleep to avoid memory issues.

Control of stress: Stress is a big memory sapper. Pay attention to your stress level whether you're having trouble focusing or recalling everyday things. Even short-term stress has been shown to affect learning and memory, according to research. Divorce, illness, raising children, and elderly parents are only a few of the issues that can arise during the menopause process. It is a survival skill to take care of yourself and reduce tension in your life. Memory issues may be an early warning sign that the stress level is rising.

Weight Gain

For women over 50, weight gain is often a source of irritation. The exact mechanism by which estrogen affects metabolism is unknown. What is obvious, however, is that many women who have never struggled to maintain a healthy weight before menopause continue to do so during and after the menopause era. Although there are no validated herbal weight loss remedies, there are lifestyle and dietary improvements that can help you naturally reduce your weight gain.

Stress management: Stress, especially the production of the stress hormone cortisol, may impair your body's ability to maintain a healthy weight.

It would be easier for your body to regulate calories and fat metabolism if you keep cortisol levels down.

Diet must-haves include: The menopause process is an excellent opportunity to review your diet and make lifestyle adjustments that will benefit you for the rest of your life. You should amend your thinking to include a good menopause diet that will set the stage for a balanced postmenopause as your metabolism slows and you begin to treat calories differently.

Everyone agrees that exercise is beneficial to one's health. However, when you approach menopause, it becomes an essential part of the overall health strategy. Weight loss, of course, necessitates increased physical activity. Exercise, on the other hand, is an all-purpose solution to menopause wellbeing since it improves memory, mood, and bone health. Exercise is the only thing that can help you control your weight to its full potential.

Sleep: You would think that getting enough sleep would sabotage your weight loss efforts, but the opposite is true. When you don't get enough sleep, it makes you want to eat more and causes your body to store fat around your midsection. A good night's sleep helps the body reset and recover from the pressures of the day. If you get enough sleep, the body can function more effectively in any way.

Cholesterol levels are high.

As estrogen levels drop during menopause, your cholesterol levels will rise. Women are soon at the same risk as men for heart disease. You can lower cholesterol levels in a number of natural ways.

Soy and red clover: Soy protein has been shown to lower "bad" (LDL) cholesterol and lower total cholesterol levels. Red clover appears to increase "good" (HDL) cholesterol while lowering triglycerides. It's possible that these plant estrogens step in to protect your heart when your own estrogen levels drop.

Whole grain oats: Including whole grain oats in your diet will reduce total and LDL cholesterol levels, lowering cardiac risk.

Melatonin: Melatonin can help raise HDL cholesterol levels without increasing overall cholesterol levels, in addition to assisting with sleep. This may be beneficial for women who have a higher risk of heart disease. If you're taking melatonin for sleep, you might notice that it lowers your cholesterol as a side effect.

Symptoms of the Vaginal Canal

Two concerns that women may have difficulty getting to their doctors are the loss of satisfaction during sexual intercourse and the beginning of urine leakage. There are a few things you can do if you're getting vaginal symptoms as you approach menopause:

Wild yam cream: Creams made from wild yam contain a phytoestrogen that, like other estrogen creams, can help relieve symptoms locally.

Vitamin E and flaxseed oil: Whether taken orally or applied directly to the vagina, the combination of vitamin E and flaxseed oil may provide some relief from vaginal and urinary symptoms. Women usually take them as oral supplements, but creams containing them may also be applied directly to the vaginal region.

Kegel exercises can help to strengthen the pelvic floor muscles and enhance intercourse sensation while also reducing urinary incontinence.

You can see results in 2 to 4 weeks if you do them many times a day.

Vaginal moisturizers and lubricants: Vaginal moisturizers operate for many days to make the vagina more elastic, and vaginal lubricants help minimize friction and pain throughout intercourse. Water-based products are less likely to cause an allergic reaction and are widely available in pharmacies.

How To Lose Weight During Menopause

Weight gain is common among women going through the menopausal process. Many that want to lose this weight can find it more difficult than normal to do so, and keeping it off can be difficult.

Part of the reason for weight gain before and after menopause is a decrease in estrogen levels.

Weight gain can also be caused by insufficient sleep and age-related changes in metabolism and muscle tone. The abdomen is where much of the weight accumulates.

While losing weight during menopause can be more difficult, many people find that there are a variety of methods that work.

Weight gain during menopause

- After a period of 12 months without a menstrual cycle, women hit menopause.
- People can gain body fat and find it difficult to lose weight during menopause and perimenopause (the period leading up to menopause).

For the following factors, menopause is related to a rise in body fat:

Estrogen levels dropping

- Weight gain is caused by changes in estrogen levels.
- In females, estrogen is one of the most important sex hormones.

It's involved in:

- physical features of sex
- maintaining bone health controlling cholesterol levels regulating the menstrual cycle
- Estrogen levels drop dramatically during menopause.

Low estrogen levels during menopause do not cause weight gain directly, but they can increase overall body fat and abdominal fat. Excess weight in middle age is linked to heart disease and type 2 diabetes, according to doctors.

Hormone replacement therapy can help to reduce abdominal fat gain.

Processes of the natural aging

Regular aging processes and lifestyle patterns are also related to weight gain during menopause.

People appear to become less physically involved as they get older. Their metabolism slows down naturally as well. These factors result in a loss of muscle mass and an increase in body fat.

Poor Sleep

Doctors also connect menopause to sleep problems, which can be caused by hot flashes or night sweats. Sleep deprivation has been linked to weight gain in animals.

The following are some weight-loss techniques for women going through menopause.

1. Increasing activity

Daily exercise is a great way to lose weight and improve your overall health.

Many people's muscle tone deteriorates as they age, and this deterioration can lead to a rise in body fat. Exercise is an essential part of maintaining muscle mass and preventing age-related muscle loss.

Aerobic activity has been shown in studies to help women lose weight after menopause. Resistance training three days a week can increase lean body mass and minimize body fat in postmenopausal women, according to another report.

According to the Physical Activity Guidelines for Americans, people should strive for at least 150 minutes of aerobic activity per week and two or three days of muscle-strengthening activities per week.

Body fat will be reduced and muscle will be built by a combination of aerobic exercise and resistance training.

If an individual isn't already involved, gradually increasing their activity levels can be easier. The following are some easy ways to incorporate more exercise into your day: doing yard work, such as gardening, walking a puppy, taking the stairs instead of the elevator standing up to take phone calls going for a walk, or getting another form of exercise at lunchtime.

2. Consuming nutrient-dense foods

People must eat fewer calories than they expend in order to lose weight. Dietary improvements are an essential part of losing weight.

All meals and snacks should be built around nutritious, nutrient-dense foods. Colorful fruits and vegetables, whole grains, and lean protein sources can all be included in a person's diet.

According to a 2016 study, this diet can help with heart disease risk factors including blood pressure and lipid levels, as well as weight loss.

People should make it a point to eat at least once a day:

a wide range of fruits and vegetables lean proteins such as beans, fish, and chicken whole grains in bread and cereals

Olive oil and avocados are good sources of healthy fats, as are legumes.

Processed foods, as well as those rich in trans or saturated fats, should be avoided. Here are a few examples:

- white bread
- pastries, such as cakes, cookies, and donuts
- processed meats with a lot of added oils or sugar, such as hot dogs or bologna
- Reduced intake of sweetened beverages, such as sodas and juices, can also benefit. Sugar-sweetened drinks have a high-calorie content.

A dietician or nutritionist may assist you in developing a healthy eating plan and keeping track of your progress.

3. Setting sleep as a top priority

It's important to get enough good sleep to maintain a healthy weight and overall health. Sleep deprivation can lead to weight gain.

Sleep disruptions have been related to aging and metabolic disruption during menopause in studies. Changes in sleep quality and circadian rhythms may have an effect on:

- hormones that control hunger
- energy expenditure body fat composition
- Symptoms like hot flashes and night sweats can also make it difficult to sleep.

Menopause-related weight gain can be reduced by focusing on having enough restful sleep.

4. Considering complementary and alternative treatments

Overall, there hasn't been a lot of well-conducted, definitive research into whether alternative medicine can help with menopause symptoms.

Although these treatments are unlikely to result in substantial weight loss, they can aid in the relief of certain symptoms and the reduction of stress.

The following are some examples of complementary and alternative therapies:

- Yoga
- Hypnosis
- herbal remedies
- and meditation

Restaurant portion sizes have risen over time, and people are eating out more, making it difficult to determine how much food a person requires per meal and per day.

Understanding the regular serving sizes of certain popular foods will aid in determining how much to include in a meal. For instance, here are some typical servings:

12 cup cooked fruit – one small piece milk or yogurt – bread – 1 slice rice and pasta – 12 cups cooked fruit – 1 cup cheese – 2 ounces meat or fish (the size of a domino) – 2 to 3 ounces meat or fish (the size of a deck of cards)

The following suggestions will assist people in controlling their portion sizes:

- Instead of eating snacks straight from the bag, measure them out.
- Instead of sitting in front of the tv, eat at a table.
- When dining out, order less appetizers and less bread.
- To weigh portions at home, use a kitchen scale and measuring cups.

8. Make preparations ahead of time

In a pinch, meal preparation and keeping healthy foods on hand will make it less likely for a person to select unhealthy foods.

Stock the kitchen with nutritious foods for fast meals, and prepare ahead of time to avoid impulsive, mindless eating. To avoid visits to the vending machine, bring healthy snacks with you.

9. Enlisting the assistance of friends and family

Having the love of family and friends is crucial when it comes to losing weight. For example, having a workout buddy can help people stay motivated to exercise.

Some people use social media to monitor their success, which may help with accountability.

10. Making lifestyle improvements

The trick to losing weight, in the long run, is to maintain healthy habits.

Short-term weight loss is more likely with fad diets, while long-term results are more likely with healthy practices such as cooking routines and daily exercise.

Chapter 9: The Rules to Slow Down Aging and Rejuvenate In 4 Weeks

You can't go to the grocery store without seeing a few tabloid stories on how to look younger. Although it's understandable to be concerned with wrinkles and sagging, there's a lot more to aging gracefully.

It's not about wanting to appear like a 20-something when it comes to aging gracefully; it's about living the best life and having the physical and mental health to do so. With the proper treatment, you, like a bottle of wine, will improve with age.

These suggestions will assist you in aging gracefully from the inside out.

1. Take care of your skin.
The largest organ in your body is your skin.

Source you can trust. It will better protect your body from the elements, control your body temperature, and provide sensation if you handle it with care.

To keep it looking and doing its best, do the following:

- When indoors, use sunscreen and protective clothing.
- Skin cancer screenings should be done on a yearly basis.
- In your anti-aging skincare routine, use gentle items.
- Keep yourself hydrated.

2. Workout
Regular exercise reduces the risk of diseases like heart disease and cancer, as well as allowing you to maintain your mobility for longer. Exercise also helps with stress reduction, sleep, skin and bone health, and mood.

The Department of Health and Human Services (HHS) is in charge of health and human services.

Adults should do the following, according to Trusted Source:

Two or three days a week, do 2.5 to 5 hours of moderate-intensity exercise, 1.25 to 2.5 hours of vigorous-intensity aerobic exercise, or a combination of the two muscle-strengthening exercises of moderate-intensity or greater that include all major muscle groups.

The following are some examples of aerobic exercise:

- swimming
- dancing

- cycling
- walking
- Weights or resistance bands may be used to perform muscle and bone-strengthening exercises.

In addition to aerobic and muscle-strengthening exercises, older adults can concentrate on activities that require balance training.

3. Maintain a healthy diet

When it comes to aging gracefully, eating healthy foods is the way to go. The American Dietary Guidelines You should consume the following foods, according to Trusted Source:

new, frozen, or canned fruits and vegetables lean protein, such as fish and beans

three servings of low-fat or fat-free dairy, such as milk, yogurt, or cheese that is fortified with vitamin D per day three servings of low-fat or fat-free dairy, such as milk, yogurt, or cheese that is fortified with vitamin D good fats

Cooking with solid fats is not recommended; instead, use oils. Processed foods, added carbohydrates, and unhealthy fats should be avoided.

To keep your blood pressure under control, you can limit your salt intake.

4. Mental wellbeing is important.

It goes a long way toward helping you live and age well to be comfortable and stress-free.

To hold the spirits up:

Spend time with your friends and family. Longevity and mental and physical well-being are enhanced by meaningful relationships and a good social network. Don't forget about your furry friends; getting a pet has been related to reduced stress and blood pressure, decreased depression, and improved moods.

Accept your age as it is. There is evidence that people who have a good attitude toward aging live longer and heal from disabilities more quickly. Aging is an unavoidable fact of life, and learning to accept it will make all the difference.

Engage in activities that you love. Investing time in things that you enjoy will only add to your satisfaction. Spend time in nature, learn a new skill, volunteer — whatever it is that makes you happy.

5. Keep yourself physically active.

Several studies have been conducted.

Sedentary behavior has been related to an increased risk of chronic illness and death, according to Trusted Source.

Going on walks and hikes, taking holidays, and engaging in group fitness classes are all good ways to stay healthy.

6. Reduce the stress levels

Stress has a wide range of effects on the body, from premature aging and wrinkles to an increased risk of heart disease.

There is a range of tried-and-true methods for reducing tension, including:

exercising having enough sleep talking to a friend 7. using calming methods such as meditation, breathing exercises, and yoga Quit smoking and limit your alcohol intake.

Both smoking and drinking have been shown to speed up the aging process and raise the risk of disease.

While quitting smoking is difficult, there are services available to assist you. Speak with a doctor about quitting smoking.

To avoid health risks, limit your alcohol consumption to the recommended Trusted Source level. For women, this equates to one drink per day, while for men, it equates to two drinks per day.

7. Get plenty of rest

Sleep is important for your physical and mental well-being. It also affects the health of your skin.

The amount of sleep you need is determined by your age. Adults over the age of 18 can strive for seven to eight hours of sleep a night. Every night, a reliable source of sleep.

It has been shown that getting enough sleep will help you:

- reduce the chances of heart disease and stroke
- reduces depression and stress
- Obesity risk is reduced
- improve concentrate and concentration by reducing inflammation

8. Discover new pastimes.

Finding new and meaningful hobbies will help you stay focused and retain a sense of purpose throughout your life.

People who participate in hobbies, recreation, and social events are happier, have less depression, and live longer, according to research.

9. Be careful of the surroundings.

Acceptance and living in the moment by concentrating on the present are central to mindfulness. Mindfulness has a number of well-documented health benefits that can help you age gracefully, including:

- improved concentration
- improved memory
- stress reduction

- improved emotional response satisfaction in relationships
- improved immune system efficiency

To practice mindfulness, consider the following exercises:

- meditation
- yoga
- tai chi
- coloring

10. Make sure to drink plenty of water

Drinking enough water keeps you routine and boosts your energy and mental performance. It's also been shown to help keep skin healthier and reduce signs of aging.

The amount of water you can drink is determined by the following factors:

- your thirst
- your activity level
- how often you urinate and move your bowels
- how much you sweat
- your gender

If you have any doubts or concerns about your water consumption, consult a doctor.

11. Take care of your mouth

Not only does neglecting your teeth age your appearance, but it also puts you at risk for gum disease, which is related to heart disease, stroke, and bacterial pneumonia.

It's important to see a dentist on a regular basis in addition to practicing good oral hygiene.

A dentist may detect symptoms of dietary deficiency, infection, cancer, and other illnesses such as diabetes, according to the American Dental Association. Brushing twice a day, flossing once a day, and using a mouth rinse are all recommended.

12. See a doctor on a regular basis.

Seeing a doctor on a regular basis will assist the doctor in detecting problems early on, or even before they begin. The frequency at which you see a doctor is determined by your age, lifestyle, family history, and pre-existing conditions.

When you get older, ask your doctor how often you can have checkups and screening tests. Often, see a doctor if you have any troubling signs.

Slow the Aging Process-in 7 Days

By taking a few small anti-aging measures every day, you can reduce the risk of diseases that accelerate the aging process while also reversing-or at the very least minimizing-damage from existing health conditions. Here's a seven-day plan to help you avoid age-related illnesses.

DAY 1 OF THE ANTI-AGING PLAN

8 A.M.
Start writing down everything you eat and drink this week in a small notebook this morning. People who maintain thorough diet diaries are more likely to lose weight and keep it off than those who don't, according to studies. Even if you don't need to lose weight, keeping a one-week food diary will show you where your diet is lacking in fruits and vegetables, healthy fats, fiber, and other nutrients that are good for you.

10 A.M
Anything with trans-fatty acids should be thrown out of your kitchen cabinet and pantry. (Hint: If the term "hydrogenated" appears in the list, it contains them.) Remove any corn, cottonseed, peanut, safflower, sesame, soybean, and sunflower oil from your pantry. Put olive and canola oil on your shopping list if you don't already have them.

1 P.M.
Place them in a basket on your kitchen counter next to the coffee maker when you get home so you remember to take them every day.

4 P.M.
Tonight, make a meatless meal. Using soy crumbles, canned or fresh tomatoes, fresh herbs, onions, garlic, and grated carrots, top a bean, tofu, or whole-grain pasta dish. Remember to start your meal with a salad; you'll eat less overall.

DAY 2 OF THE ANTI-AGING PLAN:

8 A.M.
For breakfast, combine 1/2 cup blueberries, 1/2 cup strawberries, 1 banana, 1 scoop soy protein powder, and 1 cup skim milk or soy milk in a fruit smoothie.

10 A.M
Look for yoga, Pilates, or tai chi studio in your area. Call and register for the first class that works for you.

AFTERNOON

Take a 20- to 30-minute lunchtime stroll around your neighborhood or office building. If the weather is grim, go to an indoor mall or, if your office building is big enough, walk the halls (and stairs).

6:00 P.M.

Iron-rich shrimp with sliced red, yellow, and orange peppers sautéed in olive oil and garlic with brown rice and a side salad for dinner tonight. You've just introduced another layer of defense against the six factors that contribute to aging: chronic inflammation, oxidative stress, insulin resistance, immune stress, elevated stress hormones, and toxins.

ANTI-AGING PLAN DAY 3:

8 A.M.

Scramble up two omega-3 fatty acid-enriched eggs and serve atop a piece of whole-grain toast with a side of cantaloupe for breakfast.

11 A.M.

Choose organic produce (especially strawberries, apples, grapes, and pears), free-range chicken, and naturally raised meats when doing your weekly grocery shopping (no hormones or antibiotics). Pick up two different types of fish to prepare for dinner. Place one box in the freezer and the other in the refrigerator for tonight's dinner.

3 P.M.

Take a spin around the neighborhood on the bike that has been collecting dust in the garage. Clear the debris from the stationary bike or treadmill and turn it on if the weather is rough.

10 P.M.

When you begin to unwind for bed, turn off the television and phone, put the pile of work away, and sit quietly for 10 minutes to meditate. Make your bedroom more sleep-friendly by doing the following:

- Adding room-darkening shades
- Buying a white-noise machine
- Clearing out clutter to leave a soothing environment
- Paint the walls a soothing color (such as sage green)
- Adding a small night-light so you don't have to turn on the light if you get up to go to the bathroom
- Buy new, quality pillows

ANTI-AGING PLAN: Day 4

8 A.M.
Have a cup of tea instead of coffee this morning (caffeinated is fine) and sweeten it with honey to get a good dose of antioxidants to start your day.

9 A.M.
Make an appointment with your doctor for a physical examination. It will include blood tests to check the glucose and insulin levels, as well as liver and kidney function.

3 P.M.
Get a snack in the afternoon. Remember that you're trying to eat six times a day (in small portions) to keep your blood sugar stable. A bowl of cut-up fruit and a handful of walnuts is a nice choice (antioxidants, fibre, protein, and healthy fats all rolled up into one).

7 P.M.
Take your partner or a friend to see a comedy film. Laugh a lot to relieve stress and boost the immune system.

ANTI-AGING PLAN DAY 5:
To ensure you don't have the signs of gum disease, schedule a dental cleaning and test.

10 A.M.
A glass of pomegranate juice with your morning snack will provide you with a significant amount of antioxidants.

3 P.M.
3 P.M. The probiotics in yogurt boost your immune system while also lowering toxin absorption. Flaxseeds contain blood sugar-lowering fibre and anti-inflammatory omega-3 fatty acids.

Choose these high-fibre foods to meet your daily fiber target of 25 grams:

- 1 cup bran cereal (8 grams of fiber) * 1 cup black beans (no added lard or other fat) (19 grams of fibre)
- 7-grain bread, 2 slices (6.5 grams of fibre)
- 1/2 cup broccoli, raw (4 grams of fibre)
- 1/2 cup canned chickpeas (6 grams of fiber) * 3 dried figs (10.5 grams of fiber) (9 grams of fibre)

6 P.M.

Pick up a filter for your kitchen faucet on your way home from the shop. The filter removes the majority of contaminants from your water supply, reducing oxidative stress and inflammation while also giving your liver a break.

ANTI-AGING PLAN: DAY 6

ALL DAY:

Serve yourself a little less food than normal (unless you're trying to gain weight, of course). Chronic inflammation, oxidative stress, insulin resistance, immune stress, elevated stress hormones, and toxin exposure are all contributors to aging, and losing weight is one of the easiest ways to treat nearly all of them.

5:00 p.m.

Ask a salesperson at your local wine shop to recommend a fine cabernet or merlot for dinner tonight (but just one glass—perfect it's for reducing inflammation, reducing oxidative stress, and reducing stress).

In olive oil, sauté a mixture of chopped enoki, chanterelle, portobello, shiitake, and oyster mushrooms (or any two from the list) with a garlic clove. Serve over whole wheat pasta to reap the immune-boosting advantages of the mushrooms.

10 P.M.

To improve the detoxification system, take two probiotic capsules before bed.

ANTI-AGING PLAN: DAY 7

7 A.M.

If your doctor says it's safe, take a buffered baby aspirin with your breakfast to minimize inflammation.

10 A.M.

Create a design for your own garden by looking at gardening catalogs or websites. Container gardening can provide stress relief even if you live in a small apartment. If that isn't possible, make a plan to walk in a public garden on a regular basis for both exercise and stress relief.

Other tried and true stress relievers are:

- Deep breathing
- Positive thinking to reframe a negative situation
- Meditation
- A relaxing hobby like needlepoint, knitting, painting, or woodworking

- A walk, bike ride, swim, or other aerobic activity
- Aromatherapy
- A massage
- Yoga or t'ai chi
- A warm bath with aromatherapy oils

3 P.M.

For the first sessions, make an appointment with a massage therapist. Request a referral from a friend or your doctor, and check to see if your insurance will cover it. Massage is a great stress reliever as well as a healthy way to get rid of toxins that build up in your muscles.

6 P.M.

Make a super salad for dinner tonight and you'll get almost all of your regular fruit and vegetable servings in one sitting. A foundation of raw spinach is combined with sliced mushrooms, a diced apple, a can of drained mandarin oranges, a diced red pepper, and a sprinkling of canned chickpeas in our favorite recipe. For some balanced omega-3s and immune-enhancing protein, toss in some drained, canned tuna (albacore to minimize mercury exposure) or a slice of grilled, wild salmon, and dress with mild olive oil and balsamic vinegar dressing.

How to Age Well

It is unavoidable to grow older (and certainly better than the alternative). Although you can't change your age, you can slow down the aging process by making wise choices along the way. All you eat and how you exercise, as well as your friendships and retirement plan, has an impact on how quickly or slowly your body ages.

Eat

Small improvements in your eating habits will help you avoid many of the diseases that come with getting older.

Just loss a little of weight loss

Bodyweight fluctuations may have a significant effect on health risks. It's been shown that losing only 5% of your body weight will lower the risk of diabetes and heart disease, as well as increase metabolic function in the liver, fat, and muscle tissue. That means a 200-pound individual who loses 10 pounds will reap significant health benefits. Although we'd all like to lose all of our excess weight, it's much easier to start with a 5-percentage-point weight loss target and maintain it.

Meat that has been processed should be avoided.

To maximize taste and shelf life, processed meats like hot dogs and sausages have been salted, cured, or smoked. Several studies have discovered links between consuming a lot of processed meat and poor health. According to a Harvard study, consuming one serving of processed meats per day, such as bacon, sausage, and deli meats, was linked to a 42 percent higher risk of heart disease and a 19 percent higher risk of diabetes. However, consuming unprocessed red meat did not raise the risk of cancer. Notably, it wasn't saturated fat or cholesterol that was the problem in processed meats; both whole cuts of meat and processed meats had the same amount per serving. The levels of sodium and chemical preservatives were the most significant variations. Processed meats had four times the amount of sodium and half the amount of nitrate preservatives as unprocessed meats. Processed meats have also been linked to an increased risk of colon cancer in other studies.

Blue is good for you (And Other Colors)

Though you shouldn't base your health on anyone "superfood," blueberries have a lot to offer. Eating three or more servings of blueberries a week was linked to a 26 percent lower risk of diabetes in one study of 187,000 male and female health workers. Another research discovered that eating a cup of blueberries a day reduced blood pressure. We can't just eat a cup of blueberries every day. The takeaway is to eat more darkly colored fruits and vegetables, such as blueberries, cherries, spinach, and kale. They're high in vitamins, minerals, fiber, and carotenoids. They will also fill you up, reducing the chances of bingeing on fast food.

Avoid processed foods at all costs.

The easiest way to age gracefully is to avoid processed foods and drinks. This will remove all added sugars from your diet immediately. How do you tell if a food has been processed? If it comes in a box that must be torn open, that's a positive sign. Consider chips, granola bars, junk food, fast food, frozen pizza, and other similar products. Of course, there are several exceptions to the law. By necessity, some whole, unprocessed foods that are good for you come in packets. To name a few, consider nuts, eggs, olive oil, and milk. Follow the one-ingredient law as much as possible. If a packaged food only has one ingredient (for example, ground turkey), it's probably a good option.

You'll consume a lot of fruits and vegetables, lean meats and fish, and whole grains if you stop consuming processed foods. This is basically a Mediterranean diet, which has been shown to be healthy in various studies. A quick-start guide to the Mediterranean diet is available from Harvard Men's Health Watch. If you want a different eating schedule, go ahead and do it. Both of these diets are focused on whole, natural foods that don't come in packets, whether it's a vegan diet based on the China Study, low-carb eating promoted by Atkins or the South Beach Diet, or trendy plans like the Whole 30 diet.

What are vitamins and supplements?

Study after study has appeared to refute the benefits of supplementation. Fish oil is one of the most commonly used anti-aging supplements, but several studies have found it to be ineffective. While some research indicates that vitamin B12 is beneficial to the aging brain, the majority of evidence suggests that we get enough of it from our diet. A doctor will perform tests to determine whether you have a deficiency. A fact sheet on B12 is available from the National Institutes of Health's Office of Dietary

Supplements. Vitamin D has also become famous recently, but there is no clear evidence that we need to take more of it.

In reality, according to a 2010 Institute of Medicine study, only a small percentage of people are vitamin D deficient, and randomized trials have found no advantage to taking extra vitamin D for healthy people. The best supplement advice is to put the money into a new pair of walking shoes, a gym membership, or a delicious nutritious meal with your family and other loved ones instead. Both of these things are more likely to improve your mental and physical well-being than a supplement.

Move

An active body will age more gracefully than one that is sedentary. Consider these fitness suggestions as you get older.

Intervals of Intense Exercise

High-intensity interval training isn't as scary as it seems. It simply entails alternating short bursts of intense exercise with longer periods of rest. High-intensity interval training has gotten a lot of attention from exercise scientists in recent years because it seems to help people of all ages and fitness levels become healthier. Interval running, as opposed to slow-and-steady exercise, has been shown to benefit our bodies in a variety of studies. Interval training, according to a Mayo Clinic study of 72 stable yet sedentary men and women who were randomly assigned to various exercise groups or a control group, caused cellular improvements in muscles, effectively reversing the normal deterioration that occurs with aging. It's not too late to start exercising if you haven't already. The cells of older people reacted to vigorous exercise more robustly than the cells of the young in the study.

A standard high-intensity workout lasts less than 15 minutes, including warm-up and cool-down, but several studies have shown that it provides health and wellness benefits equivalent to or greater than an hour or more of continuous and relatively moderate exercise.

Lift Weights

As you get older, weight lifting will help you retain muscle mass and build stronger bones. And the best part is that you don't have to be a bodybuilder to enjoy the rewards.

In conventional weight-training programs, we're told to start by finding the heaviest weight we can lift at one time. This is our maximum weight for a single repetition. The remainder of the program is then formed by lifting 80 to 90% of that amount eight to ten times before our affected arms or legs shake with exhaustion.

However, researchers recently compared conventional weight training to a lighter regimen. The weights were set at 30 to 50 percent of each person's one-repetition height, and the study participants lifted them up to 25 times before they were exhausted.

There was no difference between the classes, according to the researchers. Light weight lifters developed the same level of fitness and strength as heavy weight lifters. For both classes, the key was to get tired.

To maximize the size and strength of their muscles, both groups of volunteers had to reach near-total muscular exhaustion.

Strength training will also help you maintain your speed. Strengthen the muscles in the calves and ankles. Some activities are recommended by the American Academy of Orthopaedic Surgeons.

Exercise to Make Your Skin Look Younger

Exercise tends to delay and even reverse the effects of aging on your most noticeable organ, the skin, in addition to keeping the inside of your body healthy.

Most of us begin to notice a thickening of our stratum corneum, the final, protective layer of the epidermis, which is itself the top layer of our skin, about the age of 40. The stratum corneum is the visible and tactile layer of the skin. It becomes drier, flakier, and denser as it ages, as it is mainly made up of dead skin cells and some collagen.

The dermis, the layer of skin under the epidermis, starts to thin at the same time. It lacks cells and elasticity, causing the skin to become more transparent and saggier. These changes occur in the absence of any sun exposure to the skin. They are entirely due to the passing of time.

However, exercise might be able to help. Researchers looked at skin samples from volunteers aged 20 to 84 in one report. They discovered that men and women who exercised more after the age of 40 had significantly thinner, healthier stratum corneum and thicker dermis layers in their skin. Even if they were over 65, their skin had a composition that was far closer to that of 20- and 30-year-olds than that of those their age. They also discovered that recommending exercise would improve skin quality. Volunteers aged 65 and up started jogging or cycling twice a week as a form of exercise. Scientists compared before and after skin samples after three months. The skin samples had undergone distinct changes as a result of the exercise, and they now resembled those of 20- to 40-year-olds.

Remember to wear sunscreen while exercising or spending time outdoors as one of the best ways to protect your skin.

Determine Your Fitness Level

Aerobic fitness, as calculated by VO2 Max, can be used as a predictor of life expectancy. According to an American Heart Association research statement, exercise can be a greater predictor of heart disease and early death than traditional risk factors like smoking, obesity, and high blood pressure.

Aerobic fitness, also known as cardiorespiratory fitness, is a measurement of the body's ability to provide oxygen to tissues. According to the study, that process is a "reflection of overall physiological health and function, particularly of the cardiovascular system," because it is ubiquitous and necessary within our bodies.

Many previous studies have shown that having a low aerobic fitness level is associated with a significantly increased risk of heart disease and premature death and that being out of shape may pose a greater risk of developing heart disease than having a poor cholesterol profile, Type 2 diabetes, a smoking history, or a high BMI.

Think

Aging well, in my opinion, entails taking care of both the body and the mind. The majority of what we do to keep our bodies in shape is also beneficial to our minds.

Dance as if no one is watching.

Learning while traveling may be a powerful way to counteract the effects of aging by improving both the body and the mind. The neurological effects of folk dancing were compared to those of walking and other behaviors in one study.

174 healthy people in their 60s and 70s, the majority of whom were sedentary, agreed to participate in the study by undergoing tests of aerobic activity and mental abilities, including processing speed and a brain scan using a sophisticated M.R.I. system. The participants were then divided into activity classes, which included three days a week of brisk walking, a program of gentle stretching and balancing work, and a dancing group.

Men and women in the dance community met three times a week for an hour to perform increasingly complicated country-dance choreography. The cognitive difficulty was increased by having each participant learn and alternate between two roles for each dance. Brain scans of the dancing party after six months revealed changes in the portion of the brain involved in processing speed and memory.

Notably, regardless of whether they participated in the walking, stretching, or dancing intervention, almost everyone in the study performed better on thought tests. The cognitively demanding dance, on the other hand, tended to have the greatest impact on the brain, implying that behaviors that include moving and socializing have the ability to rejuvenate an aging brain.

Unleash Your Inner Artist

An aging body and mind can be inspired by art. Music, dance, painting, quilting, singing, poetry writing, and storytelling are only a few of the activities that give older people value, pleasure, and a lively sense of well-being.

The Creativity and Aging Research, a randomized study funded by the National Endowment for the Arts, provides evidence of the benefits of art for aging. The study divided active seniors aged 65 and up into two groups: action and control. The only difference in the control group's behavior was that they were required to meet with the study researcher regularly. The intervention group was assigned to a trained artist-led comprehensive community-based art program. Painting, creative writing and poetry, jewelry design, pottery, and singing in a chorale were among the activities chosen by the fortunate participants. They met once a week for art lessons and also went to concerts and art exhibitions.

Several notable themes emerged over the course of the research. While everyone in the community was clearly aging, the participants in the arts programs seemed to be aging more slowly. In general, the health of participants in the arts program improved, while the health of the control group deteriorated. They used less medicine, were less likely to fall, and made less medical visits than the control group.

Why will making art be beneficial to one's health? One explanation may be the sense of control one has when working on a project. Art projects are also sustaining in the sense that you return to them time and time again. Participants were exhilarated by the process, according to the artists who taught the workshops, and they were inspired to continue after each artistic endeavor.

So, how does this affect you? Consider releasing your inner artist if you want to boost your chances of living a long and healthy life. Make an appointment to take the pottery class you've always wanted to take. Participate in a creative writing workshop. Join a group of fellow artists and take up photography, knitting, or painting to expand your social network and share the exhilarating feeling of making art with others.

Try Meditation and Yoga

People who run, lift weights, or dance has a lower risk of dementia than those who are not physically involved at all, according to studies. However, if you are unable to engage in vigorous exercise, there is another way. Yoga and meditation on a weekly basis will help to improve cognitive skills and prevent mental deterioration as people age.

In one research, people who practiced yoga were compared to people who did mental exercises as part of a brain-training program. The yoga participants practiced Kundalini yoga for an hour each week, which includes breathing exercises, meditation, movement, and poses. The researchers chose this type of yoga because it is generally easy for people who are out of shape or new to yoga to complete the classes.

The yoga group was also taught Kirtan Kriya, a form of meditation that includes repeating a mantra and finger movements, and was asked to meditate for 15 minutes every day. Both groups invested the same amount of time in either yoga and meditation or brain preparation.

After 12 weeks, those who practiced yoga and meditation had improved moods and scored lower on a scale for possible depression than those who had received brain training. They also performed better on a test of visuospatial memory, which is needed for balance, depth perception, and the ability to recognize objects and navigate the environment. Researchers discovered that those who practiced yoga gained more communication between parts of the brain that regulate attention, implying a greater capacity to concentrate and multitask now.

Chapter 10: Exercises to do with the IF

When it comes to cultivating longevity, both intermittent fasting (IF) and exercise are essential, but should you combine the two? Let's go over what you need to know about exercising while fasting. We'll go into the advantages of working out while fasting, as well as the differences between cardio, sprint training, and weight training, as well as some easy tips on how to make the most of your fasted workouts.

Is It Possible to Exercise While Fasting?

Yes, you should exercise while fasting because hormone optimization, not just calories and exercise, is the secret to weight loss and muscle gain. Intermittent fasting has been shown to have impressive benefits on its own, but combining it with sprint training raises the benefits of both to a whole new level. When you combine the two, you'll have more growth hormones and be more insulin-responsive, which is crucial for remaining young and lean.

Many people obsess about calories in vs. calories out and are concerned about muscle loss, which can occur if you exercise without refueling. When you realize how beneficial exercising, while fast, has on the body's hormones, you'll see that fasting and exercise aren't just OK, but they're the best way to improve your health and body composition.

Is it possible to exercise on an empty stomach?

Exercising on an empty stomach is not only appropriate, but it also enhances the advantages of both exercise and fasting. This is a multi-therapeutic approach, in which the synergy between two health-promoting things increases each other's benefits to a degree that exceeds the amount of their individual benefits.

Working Out and Intermittent Fasting

Working out before breakfast is another way of suggesting you exercise while on an irregular fast. An intermittent fast is when your body goes without food for a period of time (including while you're sleeping) over a 24-hour period. The IF window starts when you take your last bite of food or drink (other than water) before going to bed and finishes when you take your first bite of food the next day.

The duration of your intermittent fast should be between 16 and 18 hours to reap the most benefits. Eat between the hours of 10:30 a.m. and 6:30 p.m., for example.

When Do You Exercise During Intermittent Fasting?

To support the body's normal circadian rhythm, the best time to exercise during intermittent fasting is typically right after waking up or shortly after. Working out (or eating) too close to bedtime has been shown to disrupt levels of deep and REM sleep, so save your workout for the next day.

You shouldn't eat right after a workout for the same reasons you shouldn't eat right after a fasted workout: hormone optimization. According to studies, waiting two to three hours after a workout before eating stimulates an increase in growth hormone, which aids in fat burning and energy replacement (sugar). A hormone change occurs as a result of adaptation to the stress caused by a high-intensity exercise. If your schedule only allows for a lunchtime workout, you can exercise during that time and then reap the hormonal benefits from not eating for two to three hours afterward.

Intermittent Fasting and Cardio

The hormonal benefits of fasting-induced exercise are linked to the depletion of muscle and liver glycogen stores that occurs when you fast. It's fine to do cardio when intermittent fasting, but the results will be determined by how fat-adapted your body is (how good it is at burning fat for fuel, instead of glucose). You should expect a slight decrease in results if you're new to fasting and exercise; it can take up to six months for some athletes to completely adapt their fitness to this new fuel source. If you're a competitive athlete, for example, and your primary objective is to improve your race results, don't turn to fasted training a few weeks before a competition.

If you're doing cardio when fasted, don't keep the fast going after the workout; instead, refill afterward.

Intermittent Fasting and Sprint Training

Sprint training, also known as high-intensity interval training (HIIT), consists of 15-30 minute bursts of vigorous exercise followed by periods of rest. Not only is sprint training time effective, but studies show that it has health benefits that aerobic exercise alone cannot offer, such as a significant increase in human growth hormone (HGH). Sprint training has many advantages, including enhanced muscle and brain power and endurance, increased growth hormone, improved body structure, improved brain function, higher testosterone levels, and reduced depression. Many of these advantages are enhanced when sprint training is combined with intermittent fasting. Sprint training is an excellent way to integrate exercise into your fasted time, and you can extend your fast two to three hours afterward to reap even more benefits.

Weightlifting and Fasting

Lifting weights while fasting is also appropriate, but you should be aware of the role glucose plays in muscle repair after a big weight-lifting session, particularly while fasted. Your glycogen reserves are already exhausted when you exercise when fasted. If your day's workout includes heavy lifting, you can do it while fasting, but you should eat a meal right afterward. Heavy lifting, unlike a burst workout session, places enough stress on the body to necessitate an urgent refeed. Lifting weights while fasted, like cardio, can reduce your strength in the short term as your body adjusts to being a "fat burner." As a result, you may want to reserve your weight-lifting sessions for after you've eaten (in which case you can fast for two to three hours afterward) and include fasted exercise on days when you do burst-style training.

To summarize everything:

Fasting while exercising is not only appropriate but also helpful for hormone optimization (which is the secret to a variety of health benefits, including enhanced body composition).

Combining burst training and intermittent fasting for a multi-therapeutic strategy will optimize the advantages of both.

Fasting may be used for cardio and weight training, but the results can suffer slightly in the short term.

To fit the body's normal circadian rhythm, the safest time to exercise when fasting is early in the day.

Unless you're doing a lot of heavy lifting or endurance cardio, fasting after your workout will also help your hormones (for two to three hours).

Essential Guide

If you're new to intermittent fasting, you might have a few questions, and one of them might be, "Can I exercise while fasting?" If that's the case, you're not alone.

It's a reasonable concern. You need the energy to exercise, and it seems that fasting can deplete your energy reserves. As a result, you might believe that skipping your workout is the best option.

Not so easy, my friend. Physical exercise will have a profoundly beneficial impact on your wellbeing if you plan it during your fasting periods.

Fasting, Exercise, and You

Physical exercise may have a significant physiological effect when done during IF. It will aid in fat burning and have an effect on how your body reacts to insulin. Exercise while fasting reduces your blood sugar, increases your body's development of human growth hormone, and boosts your testosterone levels. You need testosterone, too, if you're a woman. When you exercise hard, fat oxidation increases, increasing your weight loss potential.

Insulin Sensitivity

Insulin is a hormone that regulates the amount of glucose (sugar) in your bloodstream. But did you know that insulin often tells your body when to store fat and instructs your muscles to absorb glucose from your bloodstream and store it as fuel?

Your blood sugar – in the form of glucose – increases as you feed. Your body releases insulin when blood glucose reaches a certain amount. Insulin tells your muscle cells to take glucose from your blood and store it as glycogen in your muscles. Your body retains sugar as fat when your muscles can no longer absorb it.

Insulin resistance, also known as low insulin sensitivity, affects one out of every three Americans. It means your body has too much glucose to store as fat, but your muscles aren't getting the fuel they need to work properly.

Exercise during a fast has been shown to improve insulin sensitivity, which is a significant plus if your insulin sensitivity is in the normal range. If you're diabetic, you might find it easier to lose weight and keep your blood sugar levels in check.

More Muscle = Increased Human Growth Hormone

Human growth hormone (HGH or GH) is needed for tissue repair and regeneration in the body. It also aids in muscle development and recovery following exercise. Following a workout, the output of this important hormone will usually increase.

There is an ideal insulin-to-human growth hormone ratio that promotes good health. Exercise increases the amount of GH in your system, which tends to boost this ratio. Increased fat deposition in the body occurs when insulin levels are elevated and GH levels are low. Low GH can slow down post-exercise recovery and make it more difficult to gain lean muscle.

Exercise in a fasted state has been shown to significantly increase HGH levels in studies. Fasting for shorter periods of time does not elicit a profound reaction, but the results can still be impressive.

Testosterone Levels are Increasing

Testosterone is a hormone that affects both men and women. Men have more testosterone than women, which is why they have deep voices and facial hair. Females also contain testosterone but in smaller amounts.

So, why is having more testosterone beneficial during exercise? Since testosterone is needed for the development of lean muscle. You'll have more energy and store less body fat if your testosterone level is higher.

More Efficient fat Oxidation

Intermittent fasting will help you lose weight on its own, according to research. Exercise and intermittent fasting, on the other hand, will make it even more successful. What is the reason for this? When you exercise, your body uses the most readily available fuel source, which is glycogen stored in your muscles. The extra glycogen contained in your liver will then be used. You'll start burning fat for energy once your glycogen stores are depleted.

When you exercise after fasting for a period of time (for example, halfway through your fasting period or right before your eating window), your body has already used up some – if not all – of your stored glycogen. When there is no more glycogen to burn, your body will turn to fat for energy.

The takeaway: If your aim is to lose weight, you can see better results if you exercise during your fast. The physiological changes that occur will help you burn fat more efficiently and develop lean muscle.

Physical Activity While Fasting Has Its Advantages
The most important advantage of scheduling your workouts during your fast is the increased fat burning. According to a 2013 report from Northumbria University, exercising before breakfast will help you burn up to 20% more body fat.

Physical exercise during your fast will also help you gain lean muscle mass. You will do better if you have more lean muscle. You'll even burn more calories all day long, not just when you're working out. Muscle necessitates more energy than fat.

How the Body Reacts to IF When Used in Combination with Various Types of Exercise
In a nutshell, whether you practice them individually or together, both intermittent fasting and aerobic exercise lower blood sugar. However, certain types of exercise, such as HIIT (High-Intensity Interval Training), can trigger an immediate spike in blood sugar by causing your liver to release glycogen stored in your muscles. So, regardless of the type of exercise you use, if you have diabetes, it's important that you pay attention to your body.

Why Working Out During IF Isn't Always a Good Idea
Although there are some advantages to working out while fasted, there are also some risks.

Your blood sugar level could plummet to dangerously low levels. Exercise improves insulin sensitivity, making it easier for your muscles to extract glucose from your bloodstream. When you exercise while fasting, your muscles have even less glucose to use, which can cause you to pass out.

You might also see a drop in results, particularly if you're a professional athlete. Fasting results in either no improvement or a decrease in efficiency, according to current data. According to a new report, endurance athletes should avoid rigorous exercise while fasting.

When determining if fasting is right for you, think about your health goals. Fasting can be beneficial if your primary aim is to lose weight. If you want to gain weight, make sure you eat enough during your eating window or switch up your diet. Regardless, pay attention to any signs your body displays when you exercise and don't be afraid to consult your doctor if you have any questions.

When Is the Best Time to Eat?
When it comes to eating and working out, there is no one-size-fits-all rule; it all depends on your body, your fitness goals, and what you eat during your eating window. However, if you're doing cardio, train before you eat to maximize its fat-burning ability, and save your HIIT workout for 1–2 hours after you eat to get the best results.

Last but not least, pay attention to your body.
Before adding fasted exercise to your program, get used to the fasting routine and don't overdo it at first. Be aware of the symptoms of low blood sugar (weakness, dizziness, "brain fog," faintness, etc.) if

you rush into an overly strenuous routine. Try a carbohydrate-electrolyte drink if you feel dizzy or faint, and lighten up during your next workout.

It's important that you remain hydrated when fasting because it's really easy to get dehydrated. Dehydration becomes much more likely when physical activity is included. Drink more water than you think you like, and avoid sports drinks until your blood sugar drops to dangerously low levels.

Is it possible to exercise while fasting? Yes, indeed. Is it necessary to exercise while fasting? Yes, but pay attention to your body.

Workouts and Intermittent Fasting

Are you a gym rat who is concerned about the impact of intermittent fasting on your workouts? Or, on the other hand, are you an intermittent fasting fan who wants to try out a gym membership but isn't sure how to go about it? When you eat in a restricted feeding window, here's a research-backed guide to sticking to a daily workout schedule – and actually maintaining results. The short version is that it's very likely, evidence indicates that it won't pose a significant challenge in terms of strength or stamina, and there are several options for making the schedule work.

We'll presume that your fasts are 24 hours or less; if you're fasting for more than a day, it's probably best not to do hard workouts during the fast.

Is it possible to exercise when on IF? Isn't it ruining the workouts?

Yes, in response to the first question; no, in response to the second! Most people can work out while intermittent fasting, according to research, as long as they pay attention to hydration, electrolytes, and total calorie intake.

Women who were doing resistance training were divided into two groups: one ate normally, and the other ate only between noon and 8 p.m. These diets were observed for eight weeks. Supplemental whey protein was provided to both classes. The researchers discovered that the women consumed about the same amount of food at the end of the 8 weeks (despite eating at different times) and that both groups experienced the same amount of muscle development. Women in both groups increased their results, with no significant differences between them. This means that IF will help you gain strength as long as you eat enough.

The participants were divided into three classes by the researchers:

Just alternate-day fasting (every other day, the subjects ate one tiny meal containing 400-500 calories; on non-fasting days, they ate normally)

Just engage in physical activity (stationary bike three times a week)

Fasting on alternate days + exercise

The third-party, which combined alternate-day fasting with exercise, lost the most weight and had the easiest time sticking to the exercise portion of the program.

For the world's athletes, this study found that intermittent fasting had no discernible impact on aerobic success in either direction.

Ramadan, the Muslim holy month during which safe adults fast from sunrise to sunset, has also been studied. While Ramadan fasting isn't quite the same as a traditional intermittent fasting program for health, the research is still fascinating. This study looked at male Judo athletes during Ramadan; the researchers discovered that the men were more tired after Ramadan and lost a little weight, but that their overall performance remained relatively unchanged. Another group found similar results in power athletes (such as wrestlers and sprinters).

Finally, all of these findings show that combining intermittent fasting with exercise is perfectly safe as long as you...

Drink plenty of water.

Make sure you have enough electrolytes.

Consume enough calories to fuel your workouts. If you need 3,000 calories for a hard training day, you can eat them all between 7 a.m. and 8 p.m., or you can eat them all between noon and 6 p.m., but you must eat them all.

How to Combine Intermittent Fasting and Workouts

Timing coordination can be a difficult task, but it isn't always as difficult as you think. So many people get tangled up in knots on whether or not they should eat before or after a workout. Actually...

It's perfectly fine to exercise when fasted — research suggests that it's not ideal for sustained aerobic exercise (e.g., a long run), but it's fine for other forms of exercise and may even cause some beneficial metabolic adaptations.

It's also appropriate to fast for a period of time after working out. Most of us have learned that we should eat right after we exercise (especially strength training) to aid recovery and ensure that our muscles have enough protein to rebuild. However, research shows that it's good to fast for a few hours after a workout before eating, as long as you consume enough calories during the day. If you're an athlete in the top 1% of your sport trying to qualify for the Olympics, improving nutrition timing will make a significant difference in results, but for most of us, the basic barometer of "I feel good when I do this" is probably enough.

With that in mind, consider the following options:

If you need to work out first thing in the morning, this is the place to be.

Work out first thing in the morning and then go without food for a few hours (your muscles won't atrophy, promise!)

Work out first thing in the morning, then eat breakfast and lunch before ceasing to eat in the late afternoon.

If you need to get some exercise in the afternoon,

Fast until 12 p.m. or 1 p.m., then have a medium-sized snack. After your first meal but before you're done eating for the day, work out halfway through your feeding window.

If you have the freedom to exercise whenever you want

Are you a college student? If you want to work from home? Are you retired? Do you have a non-traditional schedule? Choose either of the options above, or fast until 12 or 1 p.m. and work out at the close of your fasting window, right before your first meal. Some people may feel tired, sluggish, and unmotivated toward the end of their fasting window, but if that works for you, go for it!

Yes, you can exercise on IF!

It's entirely feasible, even though it might take a few tries to get the timing and logistics just right. Human bodies are extremely adaptable, so there's no need to worry about meal and exercise timing. Go for it as long as you feel good and prepared for your workouts, and you're eating enough to heal between sessions.

How to Lose Belly Fat While Maintaining Normal Hormonal Balance

Belly fat develops as our metabolism slows with age, and it is primarily determined by genetics. Another reason for belly fat? You aren't eating a well-balanced diet or exercising regularly.

Hormonal belly fat is often linked to visceral fat, which binds to internal organs such as the liver and pancreas. In comparison, subcutaneous fat is what you can pinch with your fingertips. She says it's the visceral fat that worries her because of the health issues it can cause. This form of fat, for example, could suggest or contribute to metabolic syndrome, which is a group of metabolic disorders like obesity, high blood pressure, and high fasting glucose levels, as well as diabetes.

Is there another option? PCOS, or polycystic ovarian syndrome, is a condition that affects women of childbearing age and is caused by the overproduction of male hormones. Because of their elevated blood sugar levels, they may be predisposed to type 2 diabetes. Of course, hormonal belly fat isn't always indicative of these issues. Because of hormonal changes, including a drop in estrogen during menopause, women going through menopause or IVF may also gain belly fat.

Weight-loss blocker #1: estrogen imbalance

Estrogen is a sex hormone that gives women breasts and hips while also lubricating joints. Men, too, have it, but at much lower levels. But, even in menopause, both men and women are at risk of estrogen overload, which is described as having too much estrogen in the body. After menopause, estrogen is still produced in the ovaries and adrenal glands. (Even though estrogen levels are lower after menopause, estrogen supremacy can still occur if progesterone levels are extremely low.)

Estrogen, like other hormones, is in control of how you respond to food, drink, and supplements. Simply put, estrogen superiority is the primary explanation why women, regardless of age, have a harder time losing weight than men.

How to Heal: I suggest eating a pound of vegetables per day to lower your estrogen levels (and thus help you lose weight). The fiber in the vegetable aids in the excretion of estrogen, ensuring that it does not recirculate in your body like bad luck. For women, aim for 35 to 45 grams of fiber per day (40 to 50 grams for men), but gradually raise in 5-gram increments per day to reach your target without gas or bloating.

Furthermore, consuming more vegetables will reduce the amount of meat consumed. This is important for two reasons: For starters, meat is a significant contributor to climate change. Second, over the last century, rapid shifts in industrial agriculture and cultural norms have outpaced our genes' capacity to adapt. Simply put, our DNA-driven biology hasn't yet adjusted to modern meat, and women are especially vulnerable to the estrogen-related effects of meat. There is a strong connection between meat and estrogen. Estrogen overload is more likely if you consume conventionally raised red meat.

I'm not suggesting you give up all meat for good, but there are compelling reasons to minimize your intake of traditional meat. Paleo works for some women, but not all, and I've seen men with much better results. We don't have any randomized studies on the benefits or drawbacks of consuming meat, including pastured meat. Unfortunately, there isn't enough high-quality data to say that consuming meat is healthier than eating plant-based protein, fish, or poultry.

Weight-loss blocker #2: Excess insulin

One in every two Americans is thought to have diabesity, which is a combination of diabetes and obesity. Insulin becomes imbalanced and the cells become numb to the hormone when you're overweight or skinny fat (normal weight but too much fat mass). As a result, you have peaks and drops in blood sugar and store fat because your glucose sensor is malfunctioning. Insulin isn't doing its job. Your hormones are out of whack, and you're losing weight.

How to Reset Insulin: There are a variety of ways to reset insulin, but one of my favorites is to drink filtered water with two tablespoons of apple cider vinegar. Two tablespoons of apple cider vinegar taken before a high-carb meal substantially lower blood glucose levels in people with insulin resistance, according to a 2004 report.

Of course, there are a variety of ways to reset insulin—you're certainly aware that avoiding sugar and artificial sweeteners is one of them. Remember that if your metabolism isn't working, your hormones aren't either, and insulin is the most probable culprit.

Weight-loss blocker #3: excess cortisol

Cortisol is produced in response to stress, but many of us are constantly stressed. Since I believe it is the root cause of many women's battles with the bulge, I've written extensively about it in my best-selling books. Both paths lead back to cortisol when it comes to hormone deficiency and weight gain.

Most of us are aware that cortisol overload is harmful to our appearance and mental health, but this information is rarely put into effect. All those stress hormones wreak havoc on your body over time, causing you to store fat—especially visceral fat, the most dangerous form of fat—in your abdomen.

High cortisol levels have also been related to food addiction and sugar cravings, causing you to overeat unhealthy foods such as cookies and processed foods.

What's the end result? You gain weight.

How to Heal: To reset your cortisol, you must put your caffeine consumption on hold. Over the next week, gradually reduce your caffeine intake and see how your sleep and stress levels increase.

Go from coffee to half-caffeine first. After that, I went from half-caf to green tea. Then, if necessary, switch from green to white tea, and finally, turn off the stove. Replace your cup of coffee with a steaming mug of hot water flavored with lemon and a pinch of cayenne pepper. Drinking one or two cups in the morning will help induce gastro-colic reflux, allowing toxic hormones to be released and allowing you to poop every morning.

Weight-loss blocker #4: insufficient adiponectin

One of the main hormones that tell your body to burn fat is adiponectin. Its function is to control glucose levels and fatty acid breakdown, and it is encoded by the ADIPOQ gene and secreted by fat cells. Some people are genetically predisposed to produce insufficient amounts of this fat-burning hormone, and as levels fall, body fat composition rises.

When it comes to weight loss resistance, the brain plays an important part, and fat tissue and the central nervous system have a hidden conversation. One of the chemical messengers in this secret communication is adiponectin, which controls inflammation and oxidative stress, two factors that lead to weight gain.

Pistachios are a good way to re-establish adiponectin levels. It astounds me how a single food intervention can have such a huge impact on hormone levels. Pistachios (20 percent of total energy) were found to increase adiponectin in a study of 60 people with metabolic syndrome. Waist circumference, fasting blood sugar, total cholesterol, LDL (the "bad cholesterol"), and high sensitivity C-reactive protein, among other biomarkers, all improved.

What else causes adiponectin to increase? Intermittent fasting is a form of fasting that occurs on a regular basis the simplest way to do an intermittent fast, also known as a mini fast, is to prolong the time you go without eating overnight. The minimum effective time without eating appears to be 16 hours for men and 18 hours for women. That means that if you quit eating at 6 p.m., you can wait until 10 a.m. for men and noon for women before eating again.

Exercise is also beneficial, as is eating monounsaturated fats other than pistachios, such as avocados and dark chocolate.

Weight-loss blocker #5: Thyroid

The thyroid gland, which regulates the body's metabolic rate and produces hormones that affect how we think, feels, heal, and perform, is often blamed for weight control problems.

Thyroid dysfunction sometimes leads to a diagnosis of hypothyroidism, a condition in which the brain fails to properly instruct the thyroid gland, resulting in inadequate hormone output. Fatigue, weight gain, brain fog, dry hair and skin, cold sensitivity, and other hypothyroid symptoms may occur.

Weight gain is closely linked to hypothyroidism. Many people suffer from thyroid dysfunction symptoms while having "normal" blood tests, which means they don't have a specific medical disorder but have suboptimal thyroid production. Though clients, trainers, and even doctors may attribute weight gain to the thyroid, the issue of hormone balance remains: Is a sluggish thyroid the cause of the weight gain, or is it just a symptom?

People with hypothyroidism can see small weight-loss benefits from medications, according to research. The benefits are seen in people whose thyroid-stimulating hormone (TSH) levels are above 5.0, which is far above the usual TSH high range of 4.0. People with TSH readings of 5.0 or higher may have a "sluggish thyroid," as higher TSH numbers indicate lower thyroid production. However, many people with low thyroid production have normal TSH levels, so medication benefits might not be available to them.

So, what's next? thyroid hormones may be a useful marker for overtraining in athletes. Thyroid markers can be elevated as a result of the high stress and/or volume of an intensive training program. Chronic life stress from too much work, too little sleep, or mental/emotional problems may have the same effect on nonathletes.

What does this imply for your customers? Thyroid indicators that are slightly out of control indicate increased stress or a lack of rehabilitation, indicating that clients are approaching the red line. The good news is that these clients are unlikely to have a thyroid gland that is broken. They must prioritize sleep, keep a close eye on their diet, and reduce their stress levels (easier said than done, but you get the point).

Exercise load should be the highest priority when it comes to exercise. Make sure the curriculum includes appropriate overload and training adaptation cycles.

Last but not least

I thought my way into a hormonal mess as I fought my weight every morning and was emotionally obsessed over the number on the bathroom scale. My mess became my message as I gently reset one hormone at a time. My biggest wish is for you to feel even more motivated to listen to your body and make the best choices possible about which foods and lifestyle changes can benefit you the most.

Many patients have actually had their weight under control and broken through weight loss resistance after learning that irreversible weight loss occurs as a result of hormone balance.

Women's weight is a major subject, and it's about a lot more than just losing weight. It's all about taking control of your life and feeling whole from the inside out. Wonderful things will happen when you are energetic, powerful, and in contact with your body. You can actually reflect on your highest hopes and aspirations, your life's intent, instead of feeling bloated and cranky, obsessed and neurotic, or guilty and self-loathing about your body. You should figure out what makes you feel the most alive.

PART TWO

Intermittent Fasting Recipes &21-Days Meal Plan

The concept of intermittent fasting (IF) is clear and straightforward: You eat all of your meals and snacks in a specific window of time during the day (say, between noon and 8 p.m.). Isn't that simple? So, if you're new to a fasting diet, you're probably thinking, "What am I supposed to consume on the diet in terms of foods?"

It's a good question, and while fasting diets tend to focus on the clock rather than the foods, what you eat for meals does matter if you want to lose weight. Many people believe that when you're eating in a smaller window of time and likely saving calories by missing a meal (say, breakfast if you adopt the 16:8 diet), you can consume whatever you want when it's time to eat.

However, if you completely ignore calories and don't consider the macronutrients you're putting into your body, you might end up eating too many calories or not getting enough proteins, fat, or carbohydrates to properly fuel your body.

BREAKFAST, SNACK, LUNCH AND DINNER RECIPES

1. KETO FAT BOMBS WITH SPICY CHOCOLATE

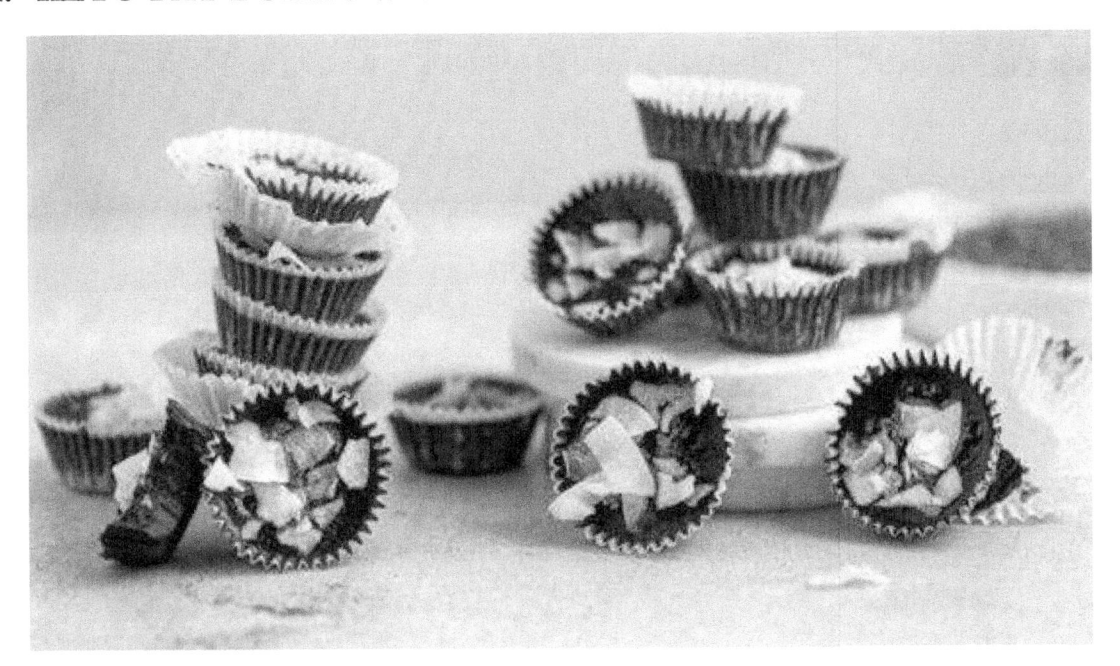

INGREDIENTS

- 2/3 cup coconut oil
- 2/3 cup smooth peanut butter
- 1/2 cup dark cocoa
- 4 (6 g) packets stevia (or to taste)
- 1 tablespoon ground cinnamon
- 1/4 teaspoon kosher salt
- 1/2 cup toasted coconut flakes
- 1/4 teaspoon cayenne (to taste)

INSTRUCTIONS

- In a double boiler set over a pot of simmering water, combine coconut oil, peanut butter, and cocoa powder. Heat, whisking constantly until the chocolate is melted and smooth.
- Stir in the stevia, cinnamon, and salt until all is well combined.

- Fill silicone mini muffin tins halfway with the mixture. (Alternatively, line a mini muffin tin with liners and split the mixture evenly between them.)
- Switch to the freezer for 30 minutes, or until the coconut and cayenne are strong.

NUTRITION INFO

Serving Size: 1 (17) g

Servings Per Recipe: 24

- Calories: 110
- Calories from Fat 93 g
- Total Fat 10.3 g
- Saturated Fat 6.5 g
- Cholesterol 0 mg
- Sodium 62.2 mg
- Total Carbohydrate 3.6 g
- Dietary Fiber 1.1 g
- Sugars 1.3 g
- Protein 2.2 g

2. Grilled Lemon Salmon

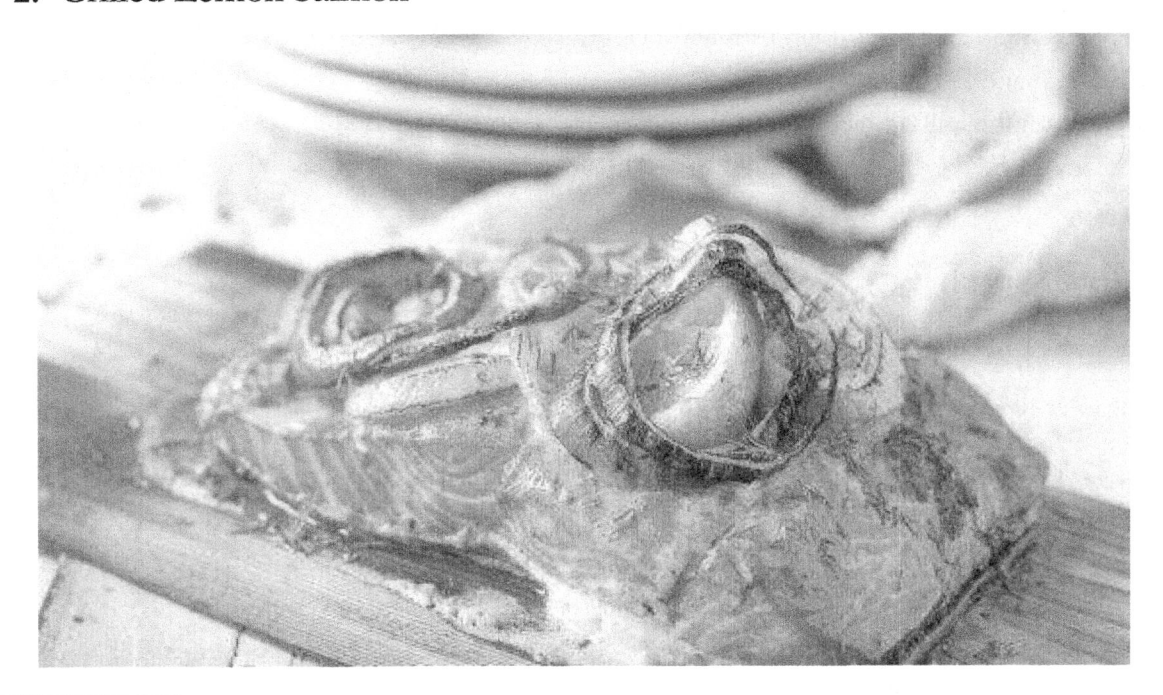

INGREDIENTS

- 2 teaspoons fresh dill
- 1/2 teaspoon pepper
- 1/2 teaspoon salt
- 1/2 teaspoon garlic powder
- 1 1/2 lbs salmon fillets
- 1/4 cup packed brown sugar
- 1 chicken bouillon cube, mixed with
- 3 tablespoons water
- 3 tablespoons oil
- 3 tablespoons soy sauce
- 4 tablespoons finely chopped green onions
- 1 lemon, thinly sliced
- 2 sliced onions, separated into rings

DIRECTIONS

- Sprinkle dill, pepper, salt, and garlic powder over salmon.
- Place in a shallow glass pan.
- Mix sugar, chicken bouillon, oil, soy sauce, and green onions.

- Pour over salmon.
- Cover and chill for 1 hour, turning once.
- Drain and discard marinade.
- Put on the grill on med heat, place lemon and onion on top.
- Cover and cook for 15 minutes, or until fish is done.

NUTRITION INFO

Serving Size: 1 (249) g

Servings Per Recipe: 4

- Calories: 380.7
- Calories from Fat 161 g
- Total Fat 17.9 g
- Saturated Fat 2.8 g
- Cholesterol 78.6 mg
- Sodium 1417.5 mg
- Total Carbohydrate 17.3 g
- Dietary Fiber 0.9 g
- Sugars 14.6 g
- Protein 37 g

3. AVOCADO QUESADILLAS

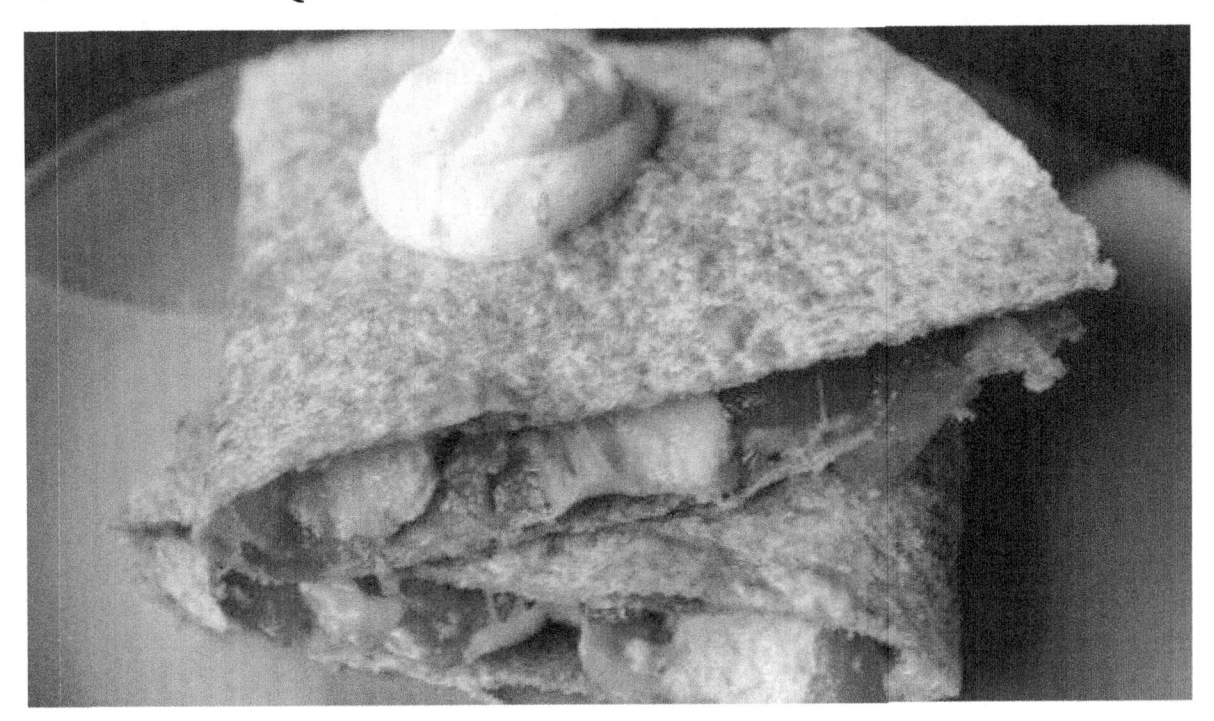

INGREDIENTS

- 2 vine-ripe tomatoes, seeded and chopped into 1/4 inch pieces
- 1 ripe avocado, peeled, pitted, and chopped into 1/4 inch pieces
- 1 Tablespoon chopped red onion
- 2 teaspoons fresh lemon juice
- 1/4 teaspoon Tabasco sauce
- salt and pepper
- 1/4 cup sour cream
- 3 tablespoons chopped fresh coriander
- 24 inches flour tortillas
- 1/2 teaspoon vegetable oil
- 1 1/3 cups shredded monterey jack cheese

DIRECTIONS

- In a small bowl, mix together the tomatoes, avocado, onion, lemon juice, and Tabasco.
- Season to taste with salt and pepper.
- In another small bowl, mix together sour cream, coriander, salt, and pepper to taste.
- Put tortillas on a baking sheet and brush tops with oil.

- Broil tortillas 2 to 4 inches from heat until pale golden.
- Sprinkle tortillas evenly with cheese and broil until cheese is melted.
- Spread avocado mixture evenly over 2 tortillas and top each with 1 of remaining tortillas, cheese side down to make 2 quesadillas.
- Transfer quesadillas to a cutting board and cut into 4 wedges.
- Top each wedge with a dollop of the sour cream mixture and serve warm.

NUTRITION INFO

Serving Size: 1 (425) g

Servings Per Recipe: 2

- Calories: 794.9
- Calories from Fat 460 g
- Total Fat 51.1 g
- Saturated Fat 21.6 g
- Cholesterol 82 mg
- Sodium 978.8 mg
- Total Carbohydrate 58.7 g
- Dietary Fiber 11 g
- Sugars 7.2 g
- Protein 29.2 g

4. VEGGIE PACKED CHEESY CHICKEN SALAD (REDUCED FAT)

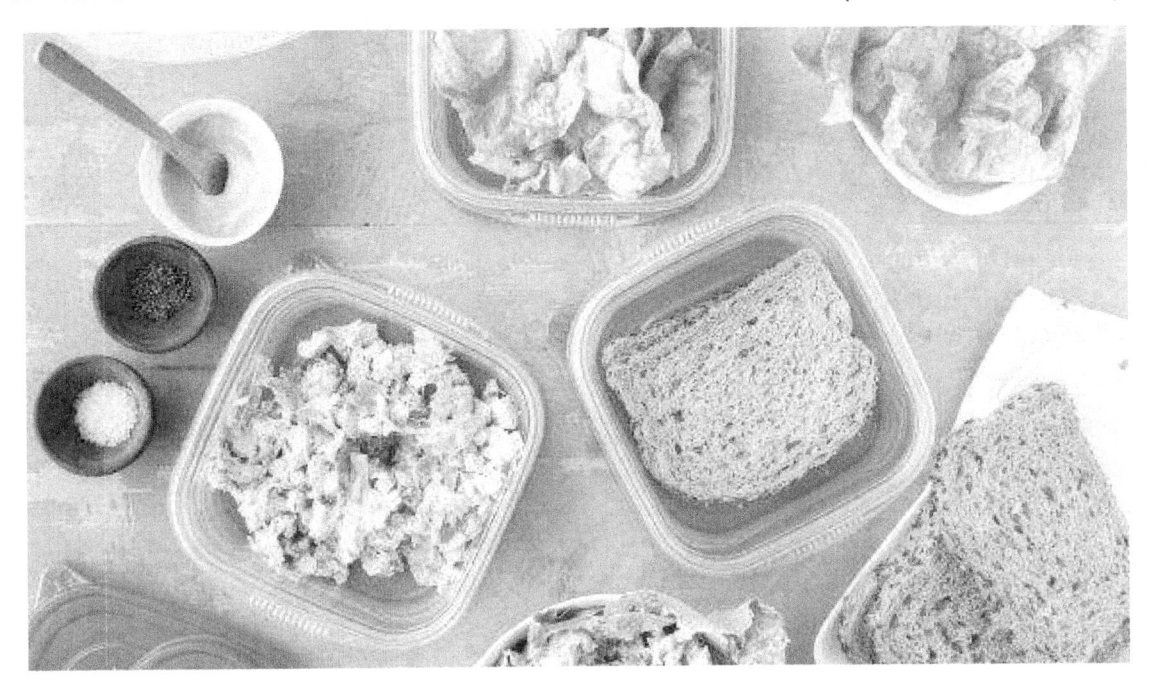

INGREDIENTS

- 1 cup cooked boneless skinless chicken breast, cubed
- 1/4 cup celery, finely chopped
- 1/4 cup carrot, shaved into ribbons
- 1/2 cup Baby Spinach, roughly chopped
- 2 1/2 tablespoons fat-free mayonnaise
- 2 tablespoons nonfat sour cream
- 1/8 teaspoon dried parsley
- 2 teaspoons Dijon mustard
- 1/4 cup reduced-fat sharp cheddar cheese, shredded

DIRECTIONS

- Mix all ingredients in a bowl so that everything is coated well with the mayonnaise mixture.
- Chill in the fridge for at least 30 minutes but you could do it the night before.
- Serve.

NUTRITION INFO

Serving Size: 1 (161) g

Servings Per Recipe: 1

- Calories: 364.5
- Calories from Fat 81 g
- Total Fat 9.1 g
- Saturated Fat 3.1 g
- Cholesterol 131.8 mg
- Sodium 767.4 mg
- Total Carbohydrate 15.3 g
- Dietary Fiber 2.8 g
- Sugars 7.3 g
- Protein 53.2 g

5. COBB SALAD WITH BROWN DERBY DRESSING

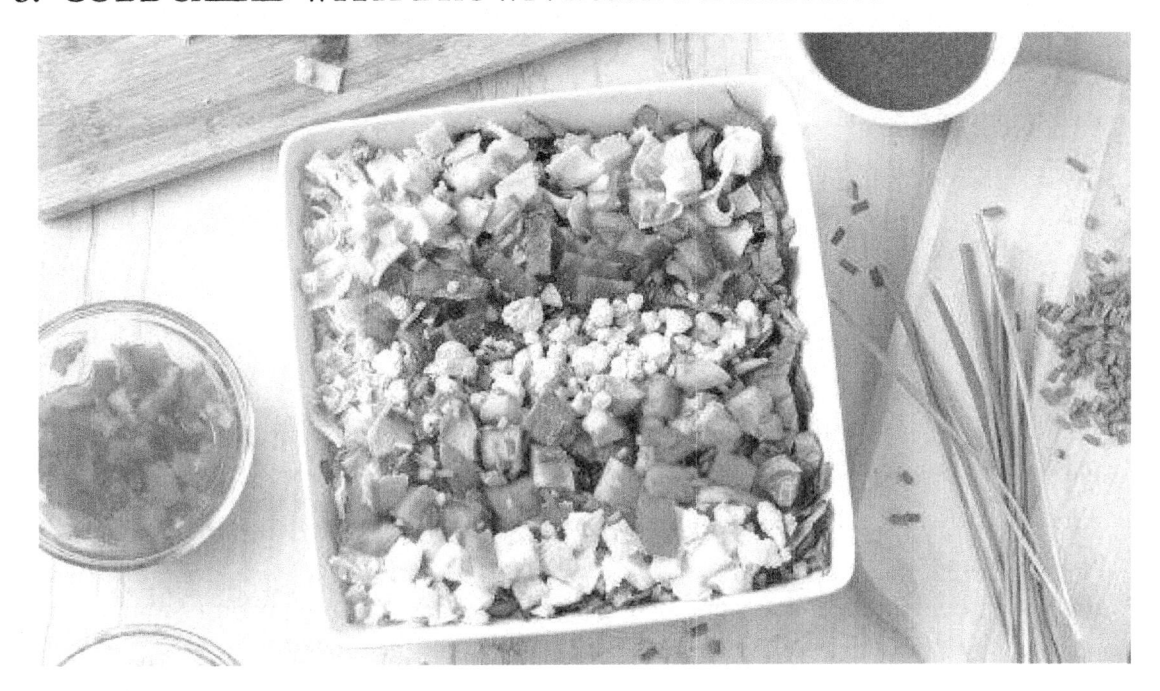

INGREDIENTS

- 1/2 head iceberg lettuce
- 1/2 bunch watercress
- bunch chicory lettuce
- 1/2 head romaine lettuce
- medium tomatoes, skinned and seeded
- 1/2 lb. smoked turkey breast
- 6 slices crisp bacon
- 1 avocado, sliced in half, seeded, and peeled
- hardboiled egg
- 2 tablespoons chives, chopped fine
- 1/2 cup blue cheese, crumbled

DRESSING

- 2 tablespoons water
- 1/8 teaspoon sugar
- 3/4 teaspoon kosher salt
- 1/2 teaspoon Worcestershire sauce
- 2 tablespoons balsamic vinegar (or red wine vinegar)

- 1 tablespoon fresh lemon juice
- 1/2 teaspoon fresh ground black pepper
- 1/8 teaspoon Dijon mustard
- 2 tablespoons olive oil
- 2 cloves garlic, minced very fine

DIRECTIONS

- Chop all the greens very, very fine (almost minced).
- Arrange in rows in a chilled salad bowl.
- Cut the tomatoes in half, seed, and chop very fine.
- Fine dice the turkey, avocado, eggs, and bacon.
- Arrange all the ingredients, including the blue cheese, in rows across the lettuces.
- Sprinkle with the chives.
- Present at the table in this fashion, then toss with the dressing at the very last minute and serve in chilled salad bowls.
- Serve with fresh French bread.
- FOR THE DRESSING: Combine all the ingredients except the olive oil in a blender and blend.
- Slowly, with the machine running, add the oil and blend well.
- Keep refrigerated.
- *NOTE: This dish should be kept chilled, and served as chilled as possible.

NUTRITION INFO

Serving Size: 1 (821) g

Servings Per Recipe: 2

- Calories: 832.4
- Calories from Fat 510 g
- Total Fat 56.7 g
- Saturated Fat 16.1 g
- Cholesterol 352.4 mg
- Sodium 3360.1 mg
- Total Carbohydrate 31.2 g
- Dietary Fiber 13.5 g
- Sugars 12.4 g

- Protein 55 g

6. MILLET & QUINOA MEDITERRANEAN SALAD

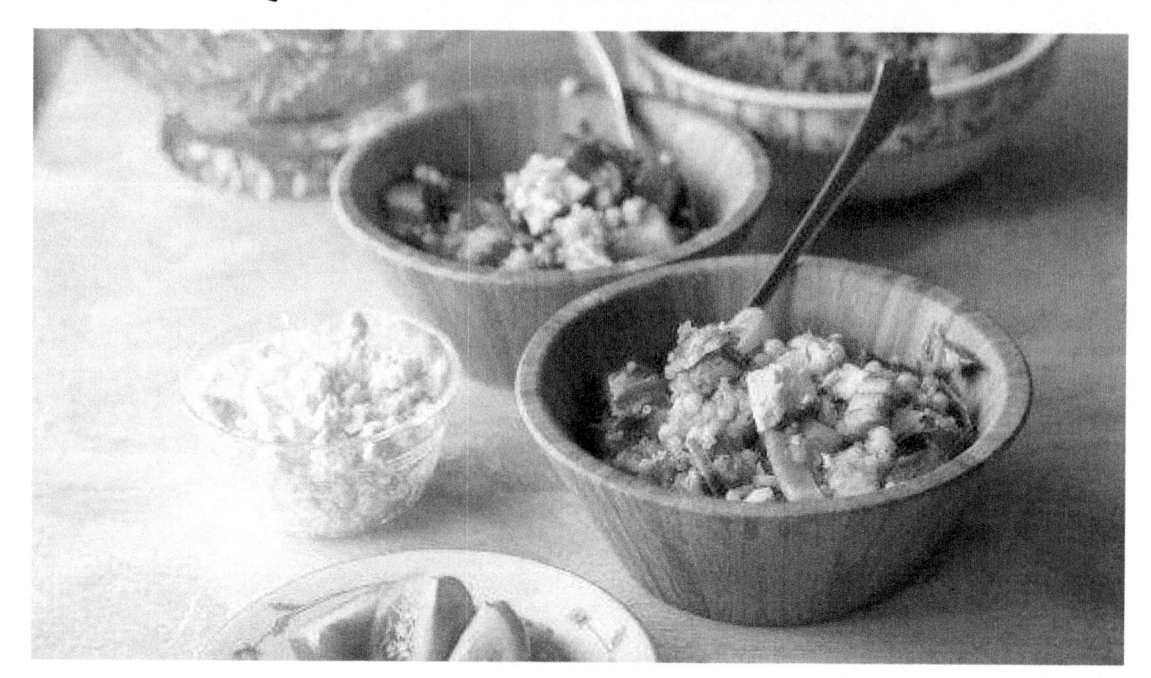

INGREDIENTS

- ½ cup millet
- 1 cup water
- ½ cup quinoa (red, white, or black)
- ¾ cup water
- 1 English cucumber, diced
- 1 tomato, ripe, seeds squeezed out, diced
- 1 sweet pepper, seeded, diced
- ½ red onion, sliced thin
- 1 garlic clove, pressed
- 200 g feta cheese, diced
- 1 (10 ounces) can large white beans, drained
- ¼ teaspoon cayenne pepper (more, to taste)
- 2 teaspoons dried dill (sub basil or oregano, if preferred)
- ¼ cup pine nuts
- 1 lemon, juice of (zest as well, if preferred)
- 1 tablespoon olive oil (optional)
- fresh ground pepper, to taste

DIRECTIONS

- Bring millet and 1 cup water to boil, reduce heat, and simmer for five minutes; turn off heat, cover, and let sit for 10 minutes.
- Bring quinoa and 3/4 cup water to boil, reduce heat, and simmer, covered, for 12-14 minutes; fluff.
- Combine all ingredients and toss; chill. Enjoy!

NUTRITION INFO

Serving Size: 1 (448) g

Servings Per Recipe: 3

- Calories: 641
- Calories from Fat 231 g
- Total Fat 25.7 g
- Saturated Fat 11.1 g
- Cholesterol 59.3 mg
- Sodium 764.6 mg
- Total Carbohydrate 78.6 g
- Dietary Fiber 12.6 g
- Sugars 9.1 g
- Protein 27.6 g

7. VEGAN FRIED 'FISH' TACOS

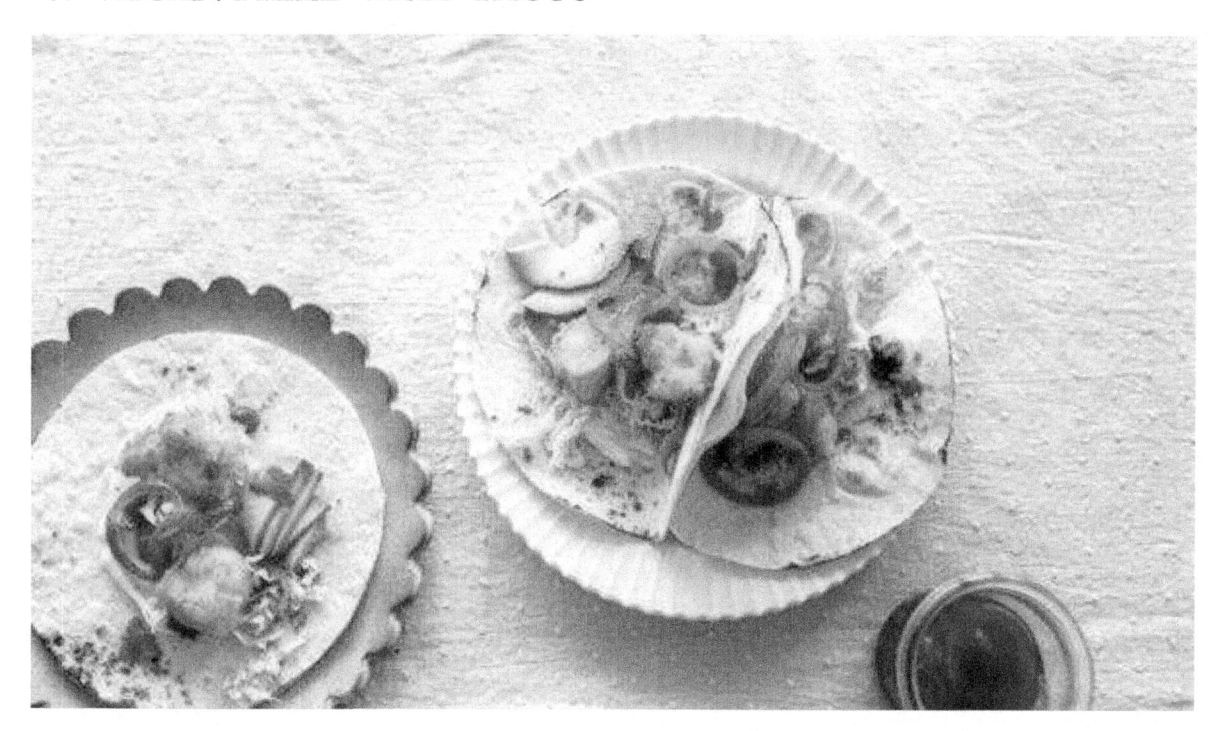

INGREDIENTS

- 14 ounces silken tofu
- 2 cups panko breadcrumbs
- ½ cup plain flour
- ½ teaspoon salt
- 1 teaspoon smoked paprika
- ½ teaspoon cayenne pepper
- 1 teaspoon ground cumin
- ½ cup non-dairy milk
- vegetable oil, for frying
- ¼ head cabbage, finely shredded
- 1 ripe avocado
- 8 small tortillas
- vegan mayonnaise, to serve

PICKLED ONION

- 1 red onion, peeled, finely sliced
- ¼ cup apple cider vinegar

- 1 tablespoon sugar
- 1 teaspoon salt

DIRECTIONS

- Pat the tofu with a few pieces of kitchen roll to remove excess moisture. Use a knife to break the tofu into rough 1-inch chunks – I like them to be imperfect, not cubes, so they look nicer!
- Place the breadcrumbs into one wide shallow bowl.
- Place the flour, salt, smoked paprika, cayenne, and cumin into another wide shallow bowl and stir together.
- Place the milk into a third wide shallow bowl.
- Take the chunks of tofu and gently coat them in the flour then the milk then the breadcrumbs and onto a baking sheet.
- Fill a deep frying pan with 1/2-inch depth of vegetable oil. Place over medium heat and let the oil get hot – sprinkle a breadcrumb in and if it starts to bubble and brown, the oil is hot enough. Add chunks of breaded tofu to the oil and fry until golden underneath then flip and cook so it's golden all over. Remove to a baking sheet lined with kitchen roll to drain. Repeat with the remaining tofu.
- For the pickled onion:
- Heat the apple cider vinegar, salt, and sugar in a small pot until steaming. Place the finely sliced red onion in a bowl or jar and pour the hot vinegar over. Let it sit for at least 30 minutes to soften and turn pink.
- Serve the hot fried tofu in warmed tortillas (I warm them over the lit gas ring of my stove), pickled onion, a smear of vegan mayo, some avocado, and shredded cabbage.

NUTRITION INFO

Serving Size: 1 (1805) g

Servings Per Recipe: 1

- Calories: 378.3
- Calories from Fat 97 g
- Total Fat 10.8 g
- Saturated Fat 2.3 g
- Cholesterol 2.1 mg
- Sodium 944.8 mg
- Total Carbohydrate 58.2 g
- Dietary Fiber 5.7 g

- Sugars 6.5 g
- Protein 12.2 g

8. MEDITERRANEAN CHICKEN BREASTS WITH AVOCADO TAPENADE

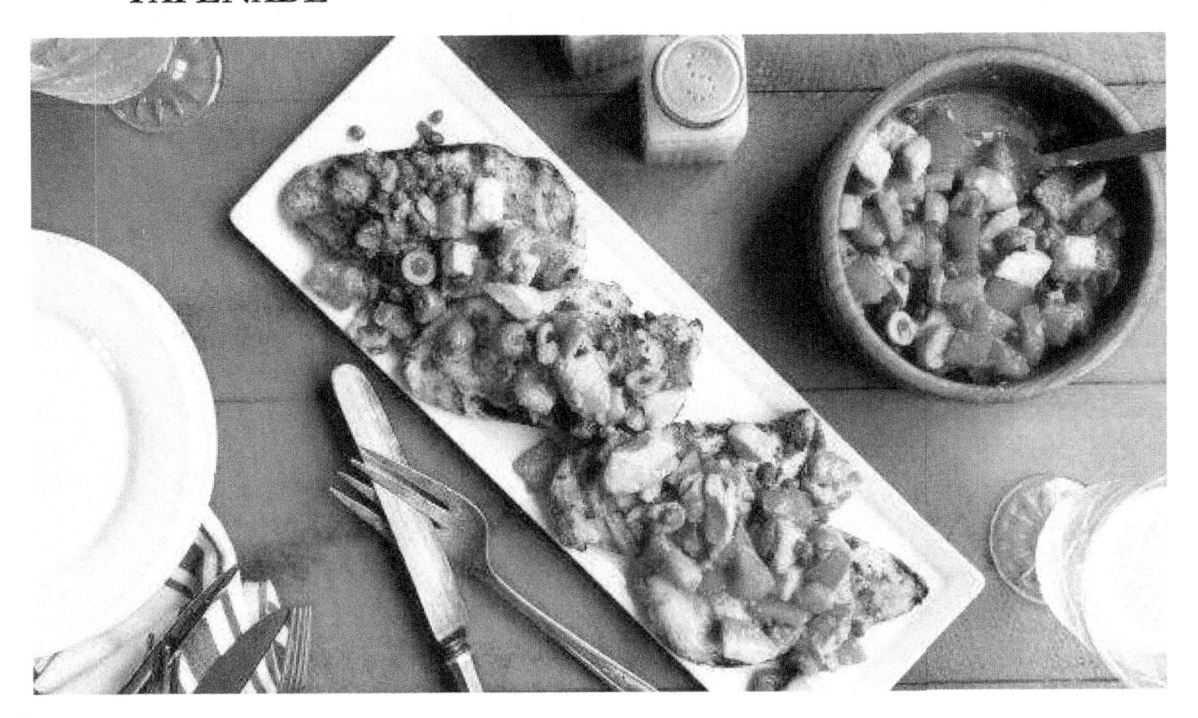

INGREDIENTS

- 4 boneless skinless chicken breast halves
- 1 tablespoon grated lemon peel
- 5 tablespoons fresh lemon juice, divided
- 2 tablespoons olive oil, divided
- 1 teaspoon olive oil, divided
- 1 garlic clove, finely chopped
- ½ teaspoon salt
- ¼ teaspoon ground black pepper
- 2 garlic cloves, roasted and mashed
- ½ teaspoon sea salt
- ¼ teaspoon fresh ground pepper
- 1 medium tomato, seeded and finely chopped
- ¼ cup small green pimento-stuffed olive, thinly sliced
- 3 tablespoons capers, rinsed
- 2 tablespoons fresh basil leaves, finely sliced
- 1 large Hass avocado, ripe, finely chopped

DIRECTIONS

- In a sealable plastic bag, combine chicken and marinade of lemon peel, 2 tablespoons lemon juice, 2 tablespoons olive oil, garlic, salt, and pepper. Seal bag and refrigerate for 30 minutes.
- In a bowl, whisk together the remaining 3 tablespoons lemon juice, roasted garlic, remaining 1/2 teaspoons olive oil, sea salt, and fresh ground pepper. Mix in tomato, green olives, capers, basil, and avocado; set aside.
- Remove chicken from bag and discard marinade. Grill over medium-hot coals for 4 to 5 minutes per side or to the desired degree of doneness.
- Serve with Avocado Tapenade.

9. SUPPER CLUB TILAPIA PARMESAN

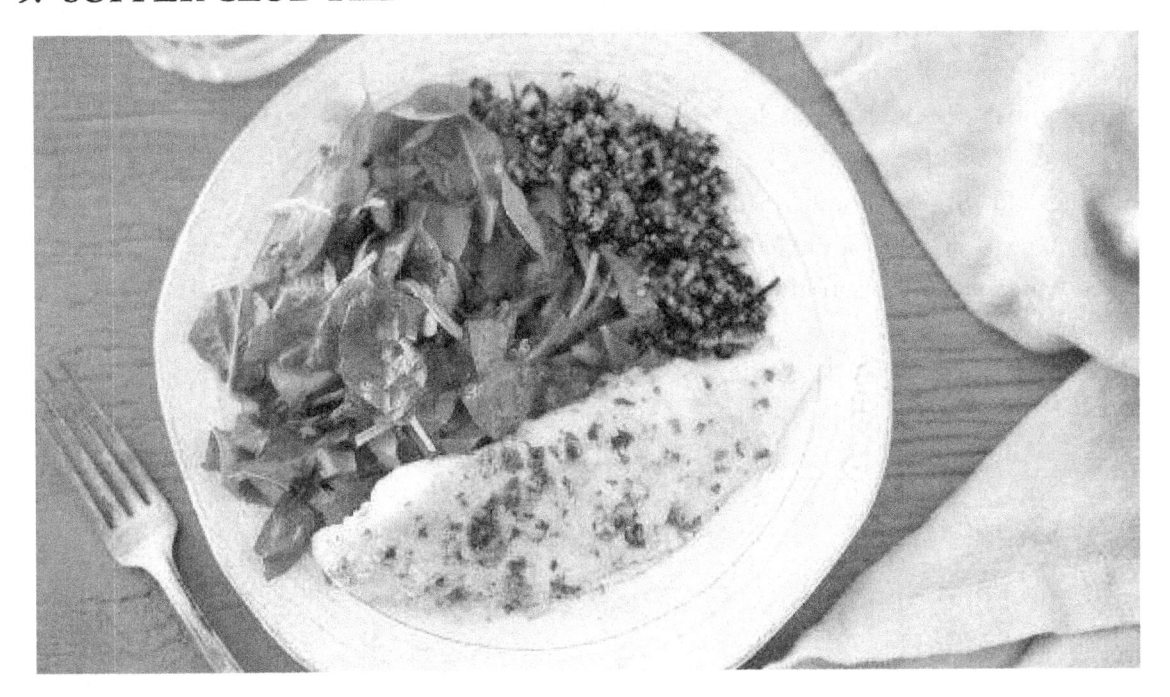

INGREDIENTS

- 2lbs tilapia fillets (orange roughy, cod, or red snapper can be substituted)
- 2tablespoons lemon juice
- ½cup grated parmesan cheese
- 4tablespoons butter, room temperature
- 3tablespoons mayonnaise
- 3tablespoons finely chopped green onions
- ¼teaspoon seasoning salt (I like Old Bay seasoning here)
- ¼teaspoon dried basil
- black pepper
- 1dash hot pepper sauce

DIRECTIONS

- Preheat oven to 350 degrees.
- In a buttered 13-by-9-inch baking dish or jellyroll pan, lay fillets in a single layer.
- Do not stack fillets.
- Brush top with juice.
- In a bowl combine cheese, butter, mayonnaise, onions, and seasonings.
- Mix well with a fork.

- Bake fish in preheated oven for 10 to 20 minutes or until fish just starts to flake.
- Spread with cheese mixture and bake until golden brown, about 5 minutes.
- Baking time will depend on the thickness of the fish you use.
- Watch fish closely so that it does not overcook.
- Makes 4 servings.
- Note: This fish can also be made in a broiler.
- Broil 3 to 4 minutes or until almost done.
- Add cheese and broil another 2 to 3 minutes or until browned.

NUTRITION INFO

Serving Size: 1 (266) g

Servings Per Recipe: 4

- Calories: 376.8
- Calories from Fat 170 g
- Total Fat 19 g
- Saturated Fat 10.8 g
- Cholesterol 155 mg
- Sodium 413.3 mg
- Total Carbohydrate 1.4 g
- Dietary Fiber 0.2 g
- Sugars 0.4 g
- Protein 50.6 g

10. SHREDDED BRUSSELS SPROUTS WITH BACON AND ONIONS

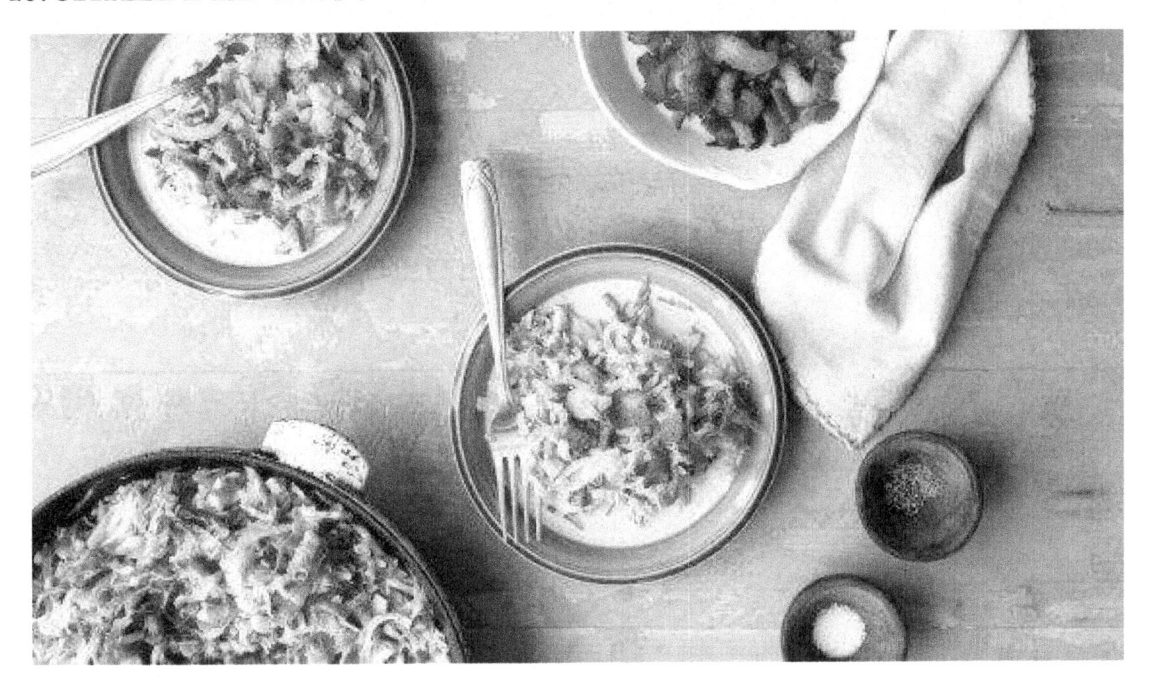

INGREDIENTS

- 2 slices bacon
- 1 small yellow onion, thinly sliced
- ¼ teaspoon salt (or to taste)
- ¾ cup water
- 1 teaspoon Dijon mustard
- 1 lb Brussels sprout, trimmed, halved, and very thinly sliced
- 1 tablespoon cider vinegar

DIRECTIONS

- Cook bacon in a large skillet over medium heat until crisp (5 to 7 minutes); drain on paper towels, then crumble.
- Add onion and salt to the drippings in the pan and cook over medium heat, stirring often, until tender and browned (about 3 minutes).
- Add water and mustard, scraping up any browned bits, then add Brussels sprouts and cook, stirring often, until tender (4 to 6 minutes).
- Stir in vinegar and top with the crumbled bacon.

NUTRITION INFO

Serving Size: 1 (123) g

Servings Per Recipe: 6

- Calories: 45.2
- Calories from Fat 14 g
- Total Fat 1.6 g
- Saturated Fat 0.5 g
- Cholesterol 1.8 mg
- Sodium 145.9 mg
- Total Carbohydrate 6.5 g
- Dietary Fiber 2.2 g
- Sugars 1.8 g
- Protein 2.4 g

11. ROASTED BROCCOLI WITH LEMON GARLIC & TOASTED PINE NUTS

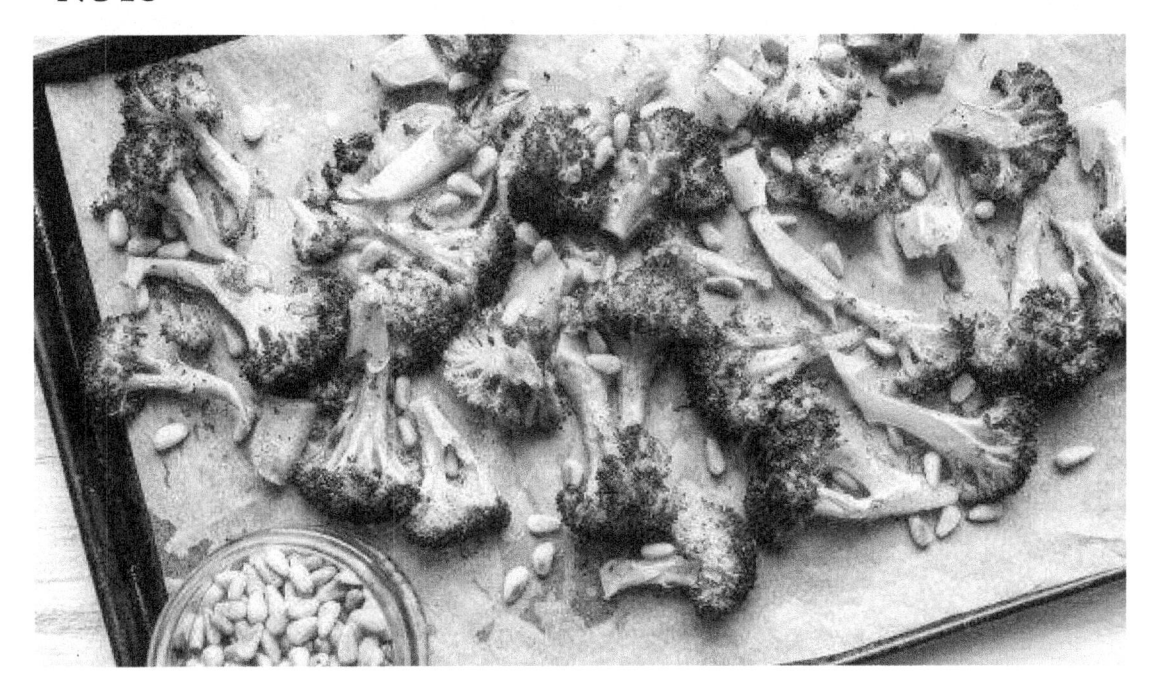

INGREDIENTS

- 1lb broccoli floret
- 2tablespoons olive oil
- salt &freshly ground black pepper
- 2tablespoons unsalted butter
- 1teaspoon garlic, minced
- ½teaspoon lemon zest, grated
- 1 -2tablespoon fresh lemon juice
- 2tablespoons pine nuts, toasted

DIRECTIONS

- Preheat oven to 500 degrees.
- In a large bowl, toss the broccoli with the oil and salt, and pepper to taste.
- Arrange the florets in a single layer on a baking sheet and roast, turning once, for 12 minutes, or until just tender.
- Meanwhile, in a small saucepan, melt the butter over medium heat.
- Add the garlic and lemon zest and heat, stirring, for about 1 minute.
- Let cool slightly and stir in the lemon juice.

- Place the broccoli in a serving bowl, pour the lemon butter over it and toss to coat.
- Scatter the toasted pine nuts over the top.

NUTRITION INFO

Serving Size: 1 (136) g

Servings Per Recipe: 4

- Calories: 172.7
- Calories from Fat 142 g
- Total Fat 15.8 g
- Saturated Fat 4.8 g
- Cholesterol 15.3 mg
- Sodium 31.8 mg
- Total Carbohydrate 7 g
- Dietary Fiber 0.2 g
- Sugars 0.3 g
- Protein 4.1 g

12. CAULIFLOWER POPCORN - ROASTED CAULIFLOWER

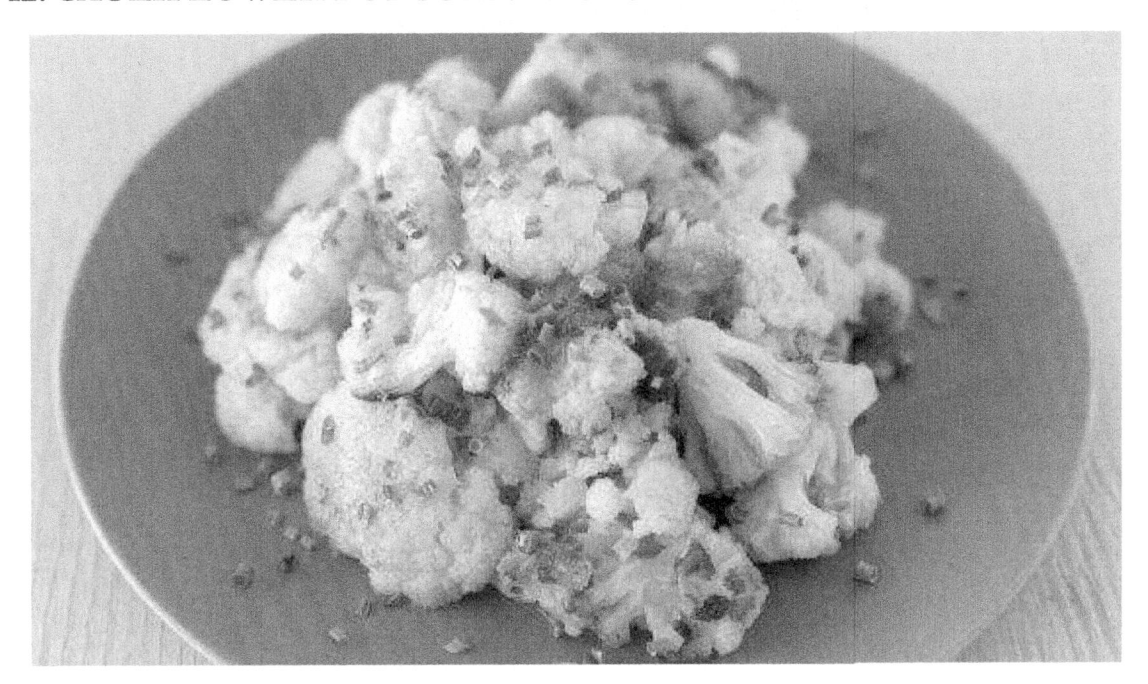

INGREDIENTS

- 1head cauliflower or 1 head equal amount of pre-cut commercially prepped cauliflower
- 4tablespoons olive oil
- 1teaspoon salt, to taste

DIRECTIONS

- Preheat oven to 425 degrees.
- Trim the head of cauliflower, discarding the core and thick stems; cut florets into pieces about the size of ping-pong balls.
- In a large bowl, combine the olive oil and salt, whisk, then add the cauliflower pieces and toss thoroughly.
- Line a baking sheet with parchment for easy cleanup (you can skip that if you don't have any) then spread the cauliflower pieces on the sheet and roast for 1 hour, turning 3 or 4 times, until most of each piece has turned golden brown.
- (The browner the cauliflower pieces turn; the more caramelization occurs and the sweeter they'll taste).
- Serve immediately and enjoy!
- Where I got it: I originally heard about this recipe at Gail's Recipe Swap, where Josh posted it and many folks tried and loved it.

NUTRITION INFO

Serving Size: 1 (162) g

Servings Per Recipe: 4

- Calories: 156.1
- Calories from Fat 125 g
- Total Fat 13.9 g
- Saturated Fat 2 g
- Cholesterol 0 mg
- Sodium 625.7 mg
- Total Carbohydrate 7.3 g
- Dietary Fiber 2.9 g
- Sugars 2.8 g
- Protein 2.8 g

13. BEST BAKED POTATO

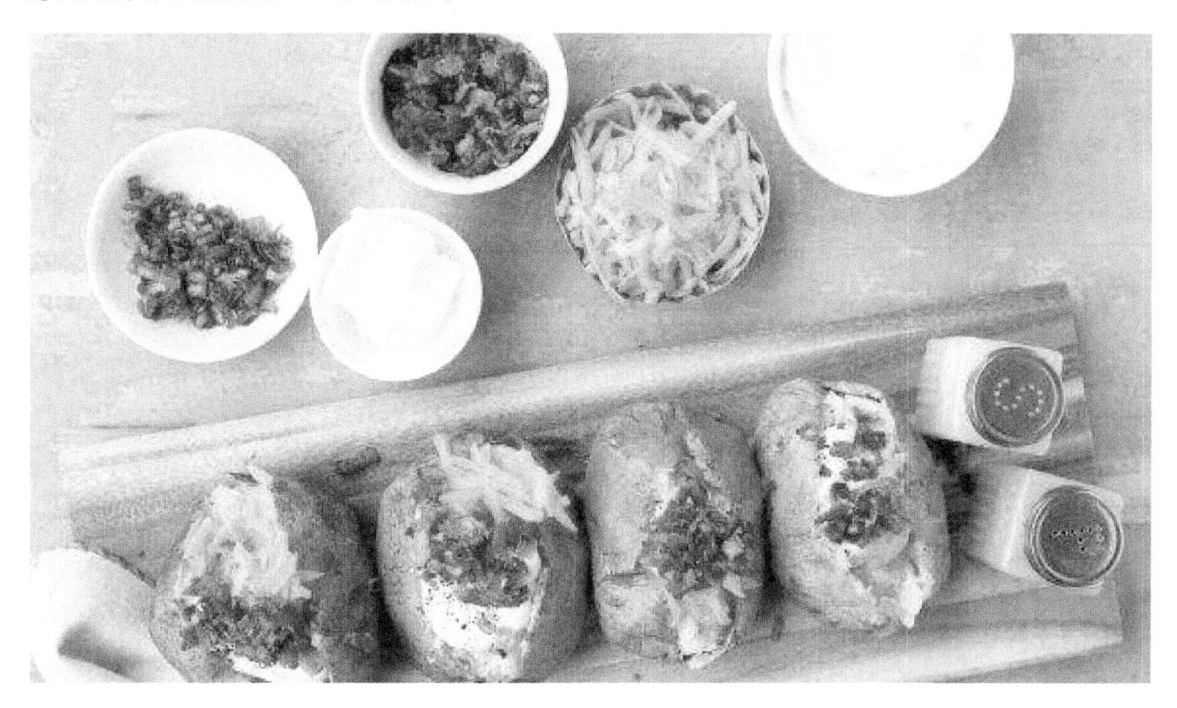

INGREDIENTS

- large russet potato
- canola oil
- kosher salt

DIRECTIONS

- Heat oven to 350°F and position racks in top and bottom thirds.
- Wash potato (or potatoes) thoroughly with a stiff brush and cold running water.
- Dry, then using a standard fork poke 8 to 12 deep holes all over the spud so that moisture can escape during cooking.
- Place in a bowl and coat lightly with oil.
- Sprinkle with kosher salt and place potato directly on the rack in the middle of the oven.
- Place a baking sheet (I put a piece of aluminum foil) on the lower rack to catch any drippings.
- Bake for 1 hour or until skin feels crisp but the flesh beneath feels soft.
- Serve by creating a dotted line from end to end with your fork, then crack the spud open by squeezing the ends towards one another.
- It will pop right open.
- But watch out, there will be some steam.

- NOTE: If you're cooking more than 4 potatoes, you'll need to extend the cooking time by up to 15 minutes.

NUTRITION INFO

Serving Size: 1 (369) g

Servings Per Recipe: 1

- Calories: 284.1
- Calories from Fat 2 g
- Total Fat 0.3 g
- Saturated Fat 0.1 g
- Cholesterol 0 mg
- Sodium 22.1 mg
- Total Carbohydrate 64.5 g
- Dietary Fiber 8.1 g
- Sugars 2.9 g
- Protein 7.5 g

14. EASY BLACK BEAN SOUP

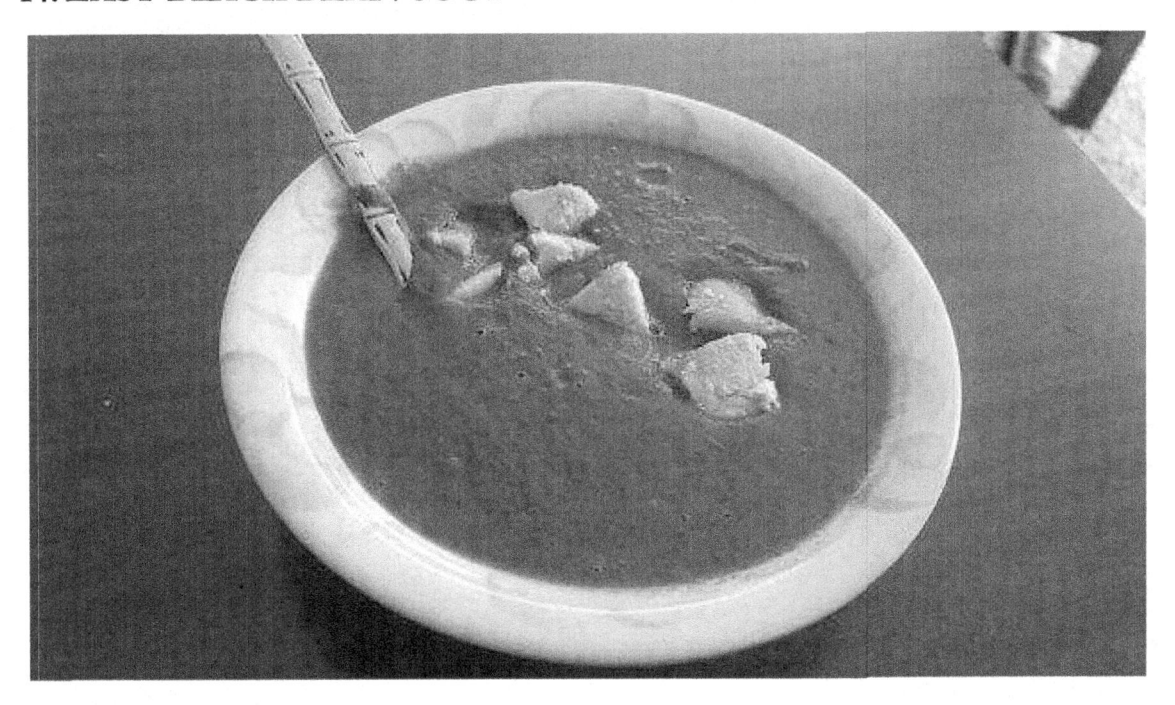

INGREDIENTS

- 3 tablespoons olive oil
- 1 medium onion, chopped
- 1 tablespoon ground cumin
- 2 -3 cloves garlic
- 2 (14 1/2 ounce) cans of black beans
- 2 cups chicken broth or 2 cups vegetable broth
- salt and pepper
- 1 small red onion, chopped fine
- 1/4 cup cilantro, coarsely chopped or finely chopped (whatever you prefer)

DIRECTIONS

- Saute onion in olive oil.
- When onion becomes translucent, add cumin.
- Cook 30 seconds, then add garlic and cook for another 30 to 60 seconds.
- Add 1 can of black beans and 2 cups vegetable broth.
- Bring to a simmer, stirring occasionally.
- Turn off heat.
- Using a hand blender, blend the ingredients in the pot, or transfer to a blender.

- Add the second can of beans to the pot along with blended ingredients and bring to a simmer.
- Serve soup with bowls of red onion and cilantro for garnish.
- I add a bit of cilantro to the pot, too.
- Can be doubled or frozen.

NUTRITION INFO

Serving Size: 1 (329) g

Servings Per Recipe: 4

- Calories: 331.1
- Calories from Fat 108 g
- Total Fat 12 g
- Saturated Fat 1.8 g
- Cholesterol 0 mg
- Sodium 380 mg
- Total Carbohydrate 41.1 g
- Dietary Fiber 13.9 g
- Sugars 2.3 g
- Protein 16.5 g

15. VEGAN COCONUT KEFIR BANANA MUFFINS

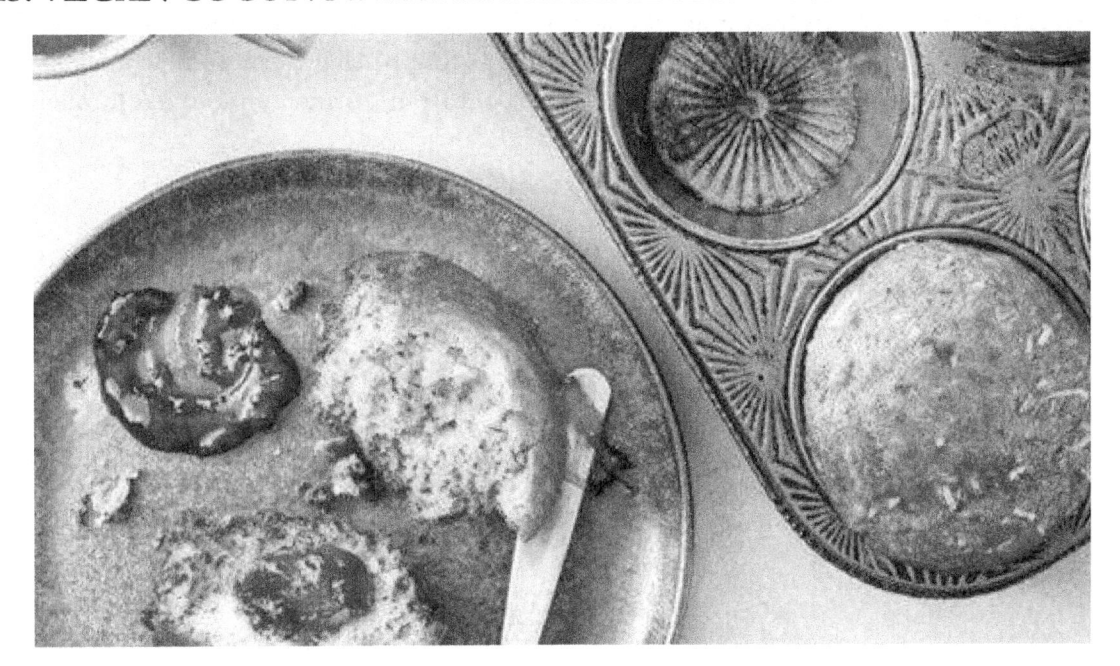

INGREDIENTS

- cups all-purpose flour
- 1 cup granulated sugar
- 1 cup unsweetened dried shredded coconut
- 2 teaspoons baking soda
- 1 teaspoon baking powder
- 1/2 teaspoon salt
- 2 ripe bananas, mashed
- 1 1/2 cups pc dairy-free kefir probiotic fermented coconut milk
- 1/4 cup cold-pressed liquid coconut oil
- 1 teaspoon vanilla extract

DIRECTIONS

1. Preheat oven to 350°F (180°C). Mist 12-count muffin tin with cooking spray. Set aside.
2. Whisk together flour, sugar, coconut, baking soda, baking powder, and salt in a large bowl. Set aside.
3. Whisk together bananas, kefir, coconut oil, and vanilla in a separate large bowl. Add to flour mixture; stir just until no white streaks remain.
4. Divide among the wells of the prepared muffin tin. Bake until tops are golden and a toothpick inserted in centers comes out clean; about 30 minutes. Let cool in muffin tin for 15 minutes.

Chef's tip: To freeze muffins, let them cool completely on a rack, then transfer to an airtight container or resealable freezer bag and freeze for up to one month. For extra protection against freezer burn, you can wrap the muffins individually in plastic wrap or foil before placing them in the container or bag. Thaw muffins in the fridge overnight or microwave straight from frozen until warmed through; about 20 to 30 seconds.

NUTRITION INFO

Serving Size: 1 (98) g

Servings Per Recipe: 12

- Calories: 300.7
- Calories from Fat 138 g
- Total Fat 15.4 g
- Saturated Fat 13.4 g
- Cholesterol 0 mg
- Sodium 344 mg
- Total Carbohydrate 39.7 g
- Dietary Fiber 2.2 g
- Sugars 19.7 g
- Protein 3.4 g

16. VEGAN LENTIL BURGERS

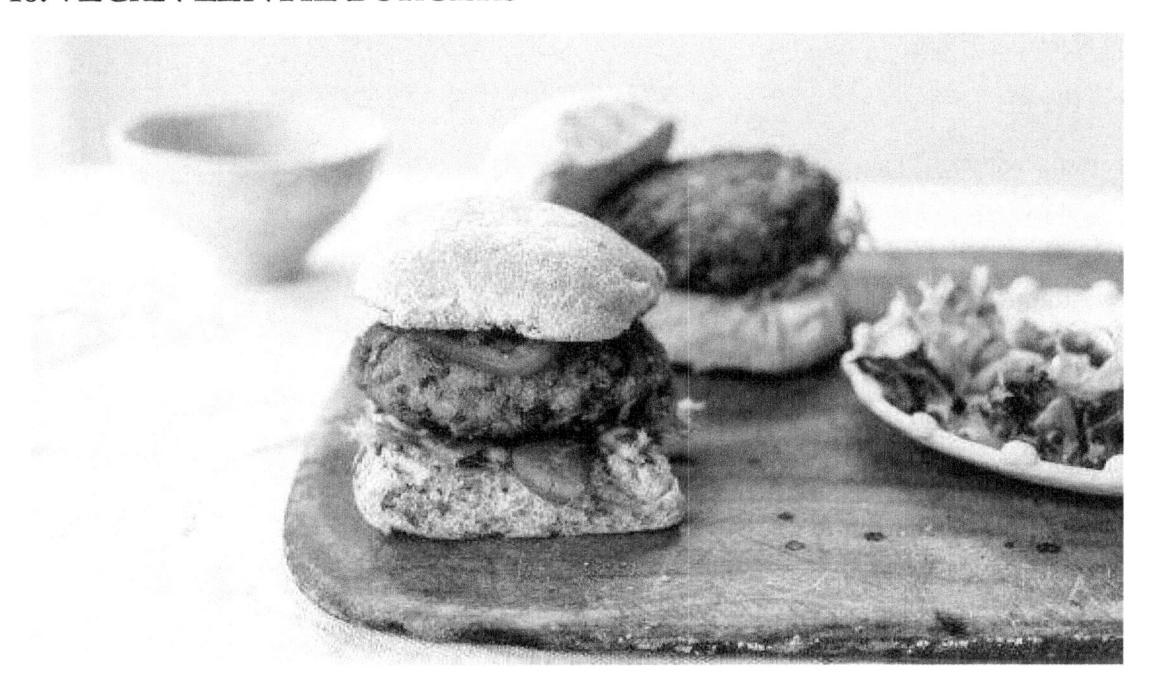

INGREDIENTS

- 1cup dry lentils, well rinsed
- 2 1/2 cups water
- 1/2 teaspoon salt
- 1 tablespoon olive oil
- 1/2 medium onion, diced
- 1 carrot, diced
- 1 teaspoon pepper
- 1 tablespoon soy sauce
- 3/4 cup rolled oats, finely ground
- 3/4 cup breadcrumbs

DIRECTIONS

- Boil lentils in the water with the salt for around 45 minutes. Lentils will be soft and most of the water will be gone.
- Fry the onions and carrot in the oil until soft, it will take about 5 minutes.
- In a bowl mix the cooked ingredients with the pepper, soy sauce, oats, and bread crumbs.
- While still warm from the mixture into patties, it will make 8-10 burgers.
- Burgers can then be shallow fried for 1-2 minutes on each side or bake at 200C for 15 minutes.

NUTRITION INFO

Serving Size: 1 (1079) g

Servings Per Recipe: 1

- Calories: 176.4
- Calories from Fat 27 g
- Total Fat 3 g
- Saturated Fat 0.5 g
- Cholesterol 0 mg
- Sodium 354.9 mg
- Total Carbohydrate 28.5 g
- Dietary Fiber 9 g
- Sugars 1.9 g
- Protein 9 g

17. SAUERKRAUT SALAD

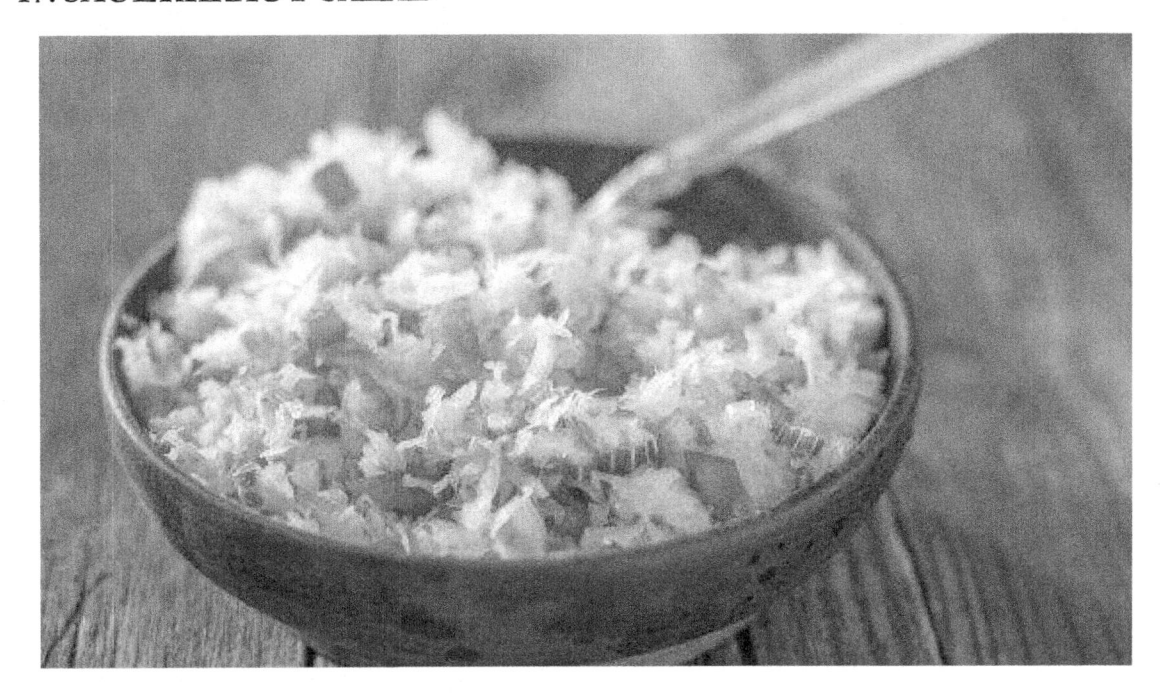

INGREDIENTS

- (1 lb) can sauerkraut, drained but not rinsed
- 1 cup celery, chopped fine
- 1/2 cup green pepper, chopped fine
- 2 tablespoons onions, chopped fine
- 1/2 teaspoon salt
- 1/2 teaspoon pepper
- 3/4 cup sugar
- 1/3 cup salad oil
- 1/3 cup cider (I use white) or 1/3 cup white vinegar (I use white)

DIRECTIONS

- Mix chopped vegetables with sauerkraut.
- Heat sugar, oil, vinegar, salt, and pepper over low heat just until sugar dissolves.
- Cool and pour over vegetables.
- Chill overnight.

NUTRITION INFO

Serving Size: 1 (145) g

Servings Per Recipe: 6

- Calories: 224.1
- Calories from Fat 109 g
- Total Fat 12.2 g
- Saturated Fat 1.7 g
- Cholesterol 0 mg
- Sodium 708.5 mg
- Total Carbohydrate 29.7 g
- Dietary Fiber 2.8 g
- Sugars 27.1 g
- Protein 1 g

18. BERRY CRISP - WEIGHT WATCHERS CORE RECIPE

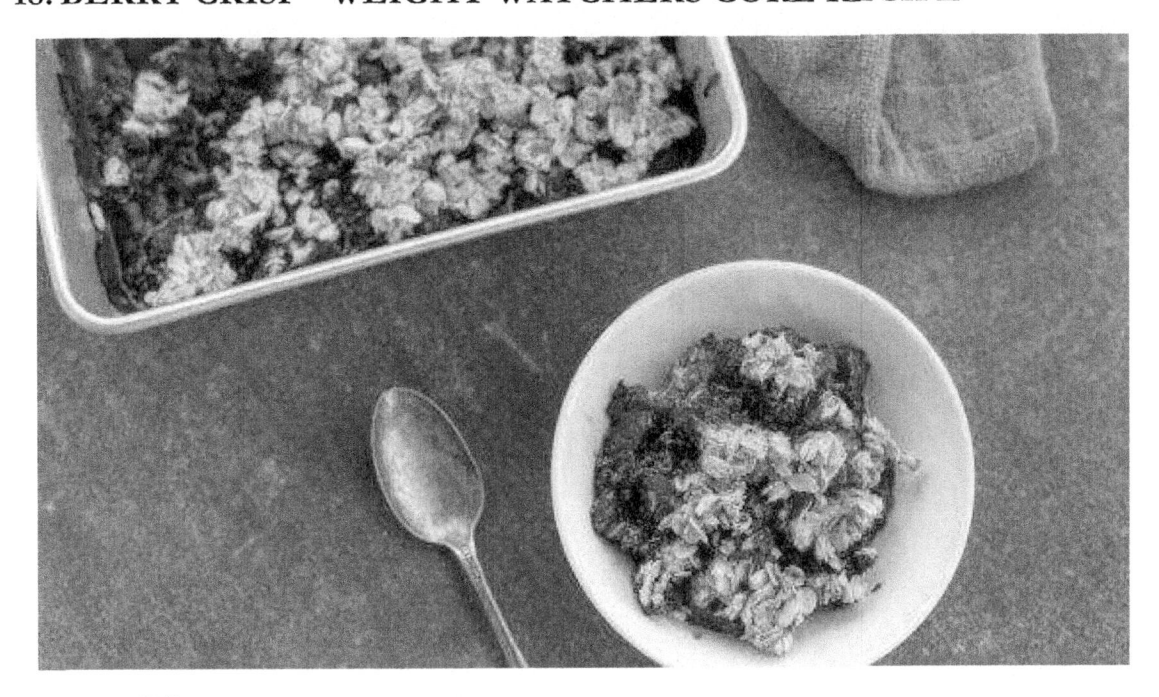

INGREDIENTS

FRUIT

- 1 (16 ounces) bag cherries or (16 ounces) bag blueberries
- 1 (7/8 ounce) box jello sugar-free vanilla pudding mix, cook and serve
- 1 teaspoon cinnamon
- ½ teaspoon nutmeg
- ¼ cup nonfat milk

CRISP

- 1 ½ cups old fashioned oats
- ½ cup Splenda sugar substitute
- 8 ounces plain fat-free yogurt
- 1 teaspoon almond extract

DIRECTIONS

- Spray an 8X8 baking pan.

- Mix the fruit ingredients in the pan and stir well.
- In a separate bowl, mix together a crisp mix.
- Spread this mixture over the berry mixture to make a top crust.
- Bake at 350°F for 40-45 minutes or until topping gets crunchy.

19. THE EASIEST PERFECT HARD BOILED EGGS (TECHNIQUE)

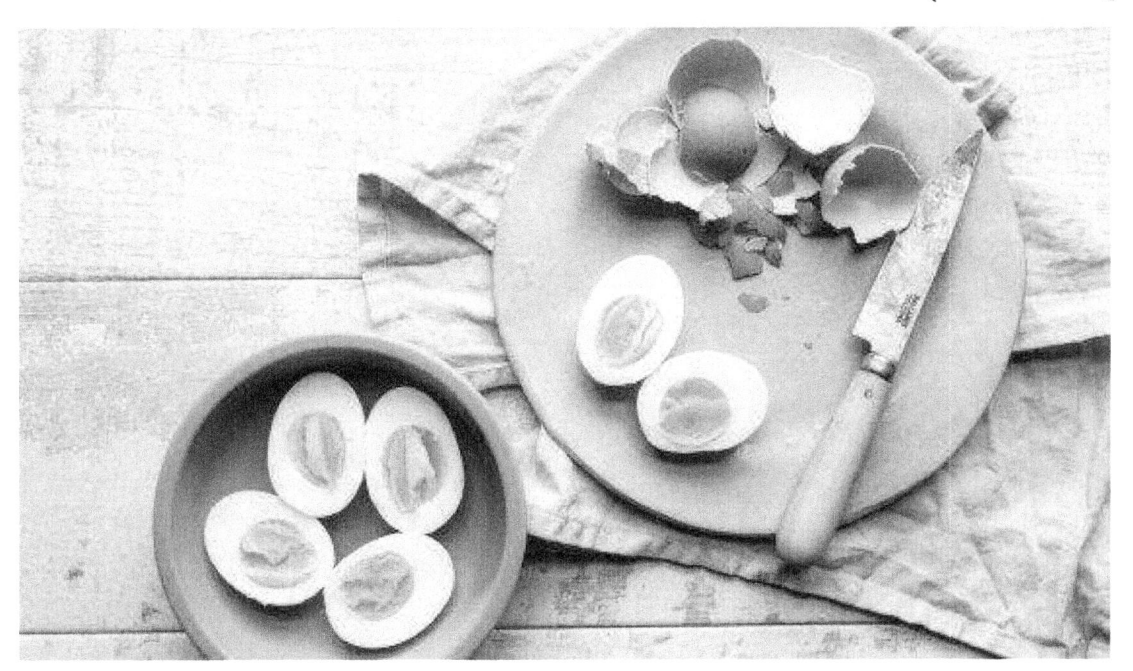

INGREDIENTS

- 6 large eggs
- water

DIRECTIONS

- Place eggs in a medium saucepan. Cover with water 1" above the eggs. Place on the stovetop over high heat.
- Bring to a boil. Immediately remove from heat and cover. Let sit for 18-20 minutes.
- Pour cold tap water into the pot allowing the hot water out by holding the pot on a slant. Let eggs sit in cold water for 1-2 minutes, then peel easily.
- NOTE: (no garbage disposal/shells for gardening method) I peel the eggs under running cold water with a colander underneath to catch the shells. I placed the eggs onto paper towels to rid excess moisture for egg salad, OR place peeled eggs into a bowl of cold water, cover and refrigerate where they keep for about 4-5 days.

NUTRITION INFO

Serving Size: 1 (300) g

Servings Per Recipe: 1

- Calories: 71.5
- Calories from Fat 42 g
- Total Fat 4.8 g
- Saturated Fat 1.6 g
- Cholesterol 186 mg
- Sodium 71 mg
- Total Carbohydrate 0.4 g
- Dietary Fiber 0 g
- Sugars 0.2 g
- Protein 6.3 g

20. TRAIL MIX

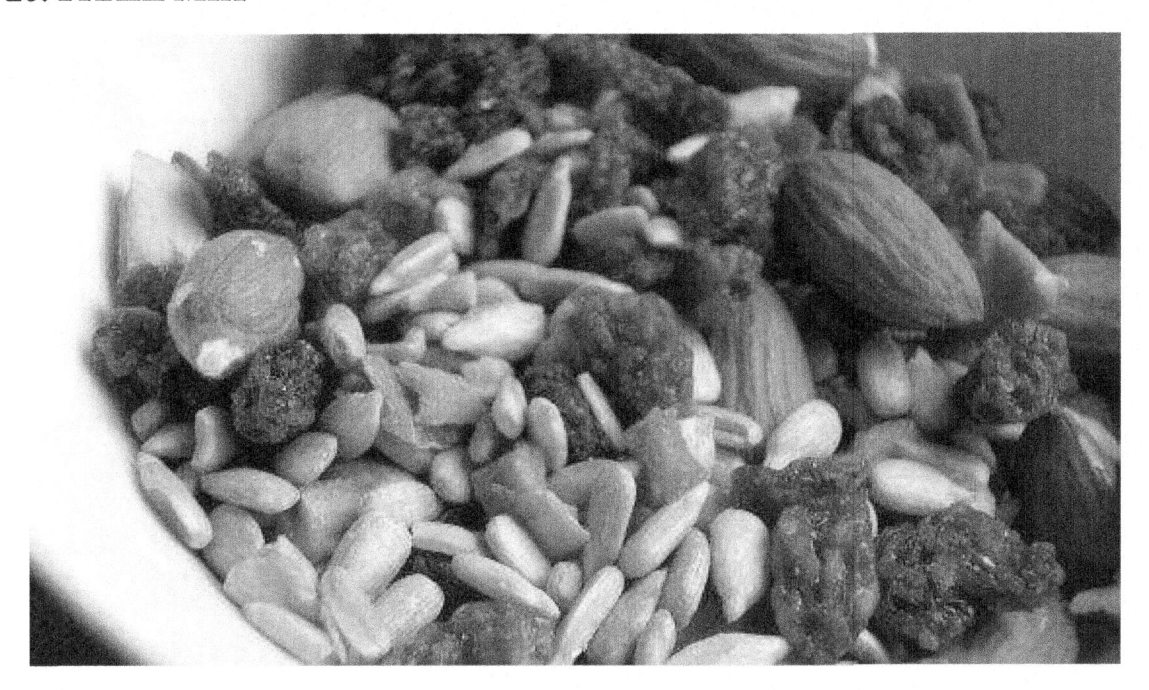

INGREDIENTS

- 1 cup almonds (raw)
- 1 cup sunflower seeds (raw)
- 1 cup raisins
- 1/2 cup dried apricot (unsulphured, chopped)
- 1/4 cup flaked coconut (optional)
- 1/4 cup chocolate (optional) or 1/4 cup carob chips (optional)

DIRECTIONS

- Pour everything into a large container, cover, and shake!
- Store in an airtight container. Place in the fridge/freezer to retain the properties of the essential fatty acids.

NUTRITION INFO

Serving Size: 1 (90) g

Servings Per Recipe: 6

- Calories: 371.5

- Calories from Fat 217 g
- Total Fat 24.1 g
- Saturated Fat 2 g
- Cholesterol 0 mg
- Sodium 83.8 mg
- Total Carbohydrate 35.5 g
- Dietary Fiber 6.2 g
- Sugars 21.8 g
- Protein 10.8 g

21. WARM ROASTED VEGETABLE FARRO SALAD

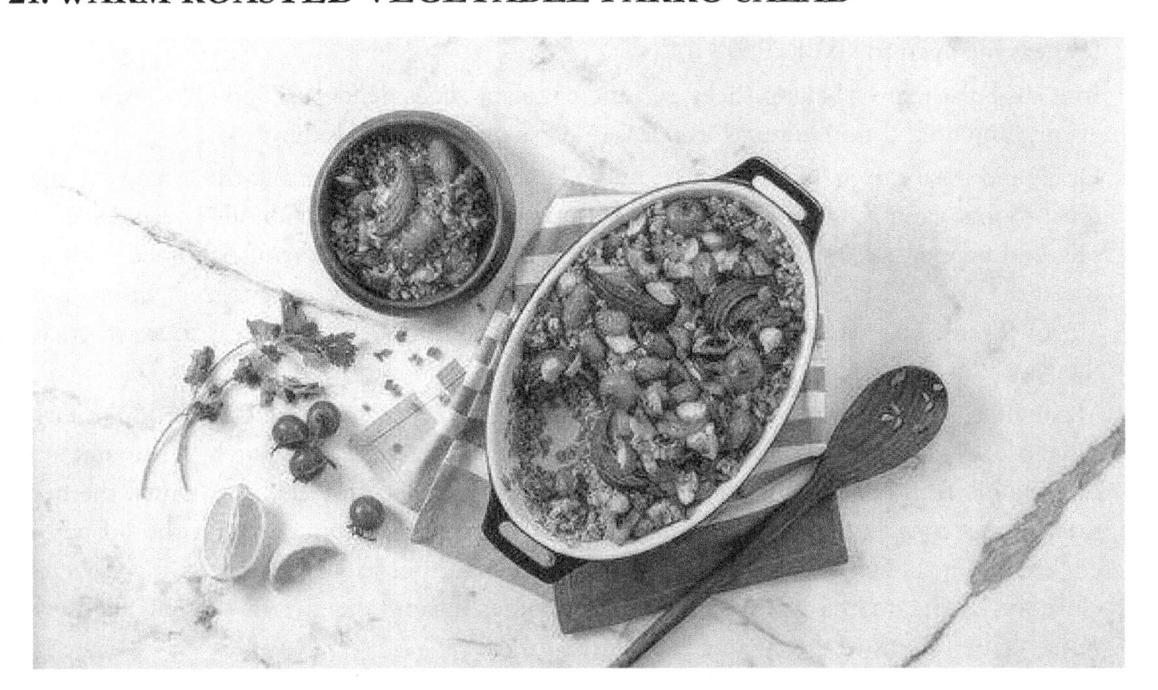

INGREDIENTS

- 1/2 medium-sized eggplant, peel on, and large diced
- 1 tablespoon kosher salt or 1 tablespoon sea salt
- 1 cup cherry tomatoes, washed and left whole
- 1 medium-sized zucchini, peel on, and large diced
- 6 white button mushrooms, quartered
- 6 garlic cloves, peeled, trimmed, and sliced
- 1/2 medium-sized red onion, peeled and cut into wedges
- 1 tablespoon olive oil
- 1 cup cracked farro
- 2 cups almond milk (Almond Breeze)
- 1 teaspoon tbsp olive oil (15 mL)
- 1 tablespoon olive oil
- 1 tablespoon balsamic vinegar
- 3 sprigs fresh cilantro
- 1/2 teaspoon salt
- 1/2 teaspoon pepper

DIRECTIONS

- Preheat the oven to 400°F (200°C).
- In a large flat pan or baking sheet, salt the eggplant slices generously on all sides, toss to coat evenly, and hold for 30 minutes to release excess moisture and bitterness.
- Drain and rinse the eggplant and toss into a large mixing bowl. Add in the tomatoes, zucchini, mushrooms, garlic, and onions. Generously drizzle the vegetables with olive oil and season with salt, and pepper, stir to coat. Transfer the vegetables to an ovenproof pan lined with tin foil. Roast the vegetables in the oven for 20 - 25 minutes or until soft, caramelized, and fork-tender. Stir or flip the vegetables about 10 – 15 minutes into the roasting process to avoid sticking to the pan. Remove the pan from the oven and set it aside.
- Meanwhile, rinse the farro with water and drain in a colander over the sink. Add the farro to a 3-quart (3L) saucepot and add in the Almond Breeze. Season with a pinch of salt and a drizzle of olive oil. Bring the liquid to boil over medium-high heat, and then turn down the heat to a low simmer to avoid spilling over. Simmer the farro for 20 minutes with the lid to the pot cocked to one side to let out steam. Turn off the heat but leave the pot on the stovetop and close the lid. Steam in the pot for another 5 minutes or until the farro is soft but slightly chewy in the center. Remove the lid and fluff with a fork.
- When ready to assemble the dish, combine the cooked farro with the vegetables in a large serving dish and gently toss to mix. Whisk together the olive oil with the balsamic vinegar and drizzle over the farro salad. Toss to coat and season with salt and pepper to taste. Garnish with fresh cilantro and a squeeze of lemon. Serve warm.

NUTRITION INFO

Serving Size: 1 (219) g

Servings Per Recipe: 4

- Calories: 123.9
- Calories from Fat 75 g
- Total Fat 8.4 g
- Saturated Fat 1.2 g
- Cholesterol 0 mg
- Sodium 2046.5 mg
- Total Carbohydrate 11.5 g
- Dietary Fiber 4 g
- Sugars 5.6 g
- Protein 3 g

22. CAJUN POTATO, PRAWN/SHRIMP AND AVOCADO SALAD

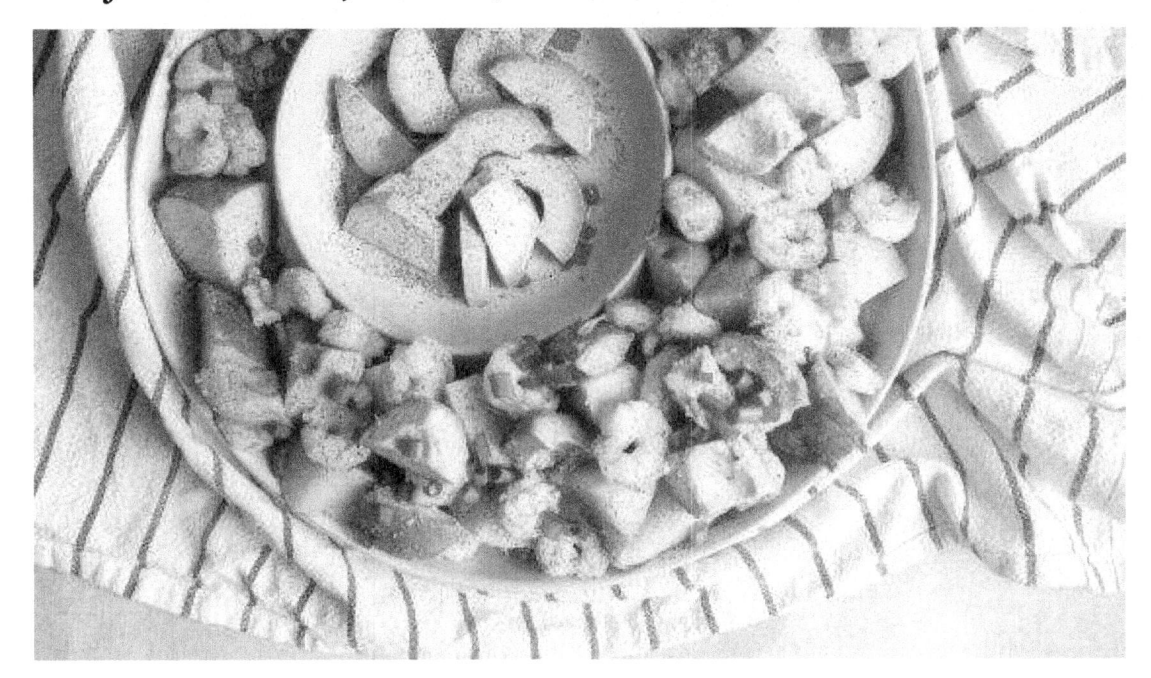

INGREDIENTS

- 300g new potatoes (small baby or chats 10 oz halved)
- 1 tablespoon olive oil
- 250 g king prawns (8 oz, cooked and peeled)
- 1 garlic clove (minced)
- 2 spring onions (finely sliced)
- 2 teaspoons cajun seasoning
- 1 avocado (peeled, stoned, and diced)
- 1 cup alfalfa sprout
- salt (to boil potatoes)

DIRECTIONS

- Cook the potatoes in a large saucepan of lightly salted boiling water for 10 to 15 minutes or until tender, drain well.
- Heat the oil in a wok or large nonstick frying pan/skillet.
- Add the prawns, garlic, spring onions, and Cajun seasoning and stir fry for 2 to 3 minutes or until the prawns are hot.
- Stir in the potatoes and cook for a further minute.
- Transfer to serving dishes and top with the avocado and the alfalfa sprouts and serve.

NUTRITION INFO

Serving Size: 1 (515) g

Servings Per Recipe: 2

- Calories: 435.6
- Calories from Fat 207 g
- Total Fat 23 g
- Saturated Fat 3.3 g
- Cholesterol 157.5 mg
- Sodium 727.3 mg
- Total Carbohydrate 37.9 g
- Dietary Fiber 10.8 g
- Sugars 2.2 g
- Protein 23.1 g

23. BAKED MAHI MAHI

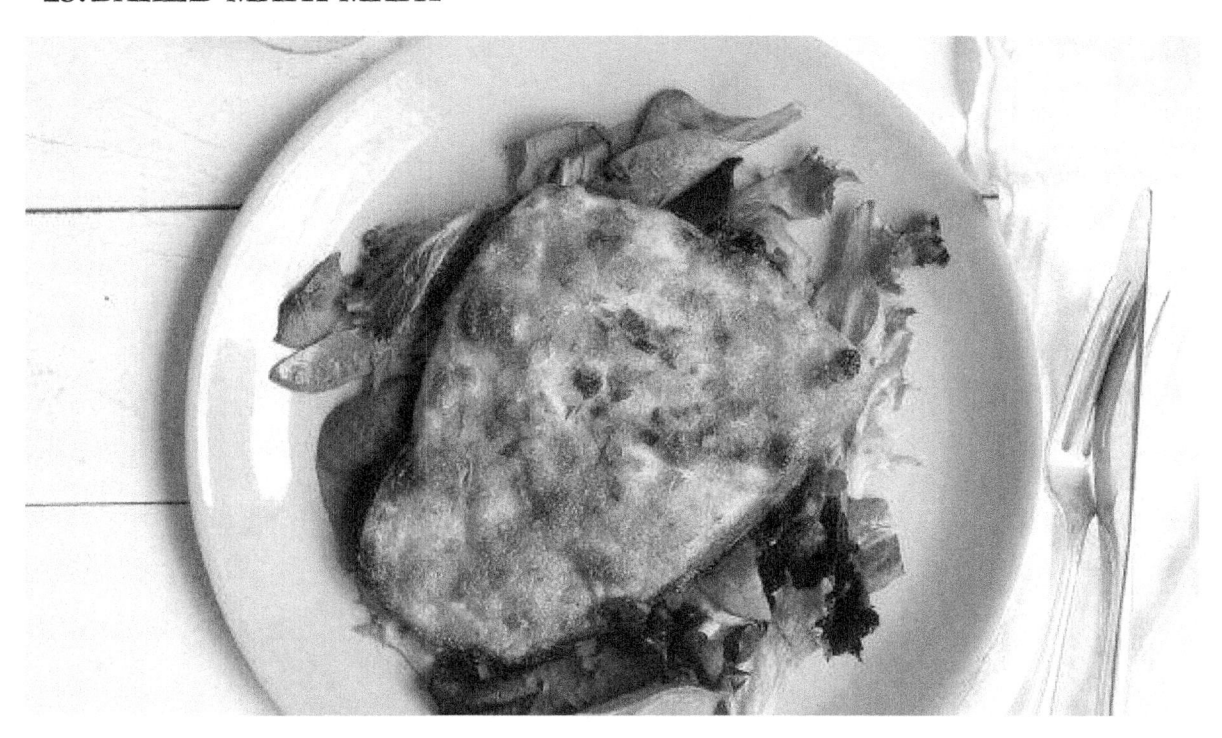

INGREDIENTS

- 2 lbs mahi mahi (4 fillets)
- 1 lemon, juiced
- ¼ teaspoon garlic salt
- ¼ teaspoon ground black pepper
- 1 cup mayonnaise
- ¼ cup white onion, finely chopped
- breadcrumbs

DIRECTIONS

- Preheat oven to 425°F.
- Rinse fish and put in a baking dish. Squeeze lemon juice on fish then sprinkles with garlic salt and pepper.
- Mix mayonnaise and chopped onions and spread on fish. Sprinkle with breadcrumbs and bake at 425°F for 25 minutes.

NUTRITION INFO

Serving Size: 1 (251) g

Servings Per Recipe: 4

- Calories: 201.9
- Calories from Fat 14 g
- Total Fat 1.6 g
- Saturated Fat 0.4 g
- Cholesterol 165.5 mg
- Sodium 200.3 mg
- Total Carbohydrate 2.5 g
- Dietary Fiber 0.6 g
- Sugars 0.8 g
- Protein 42.2 g

24. BROCCOLI DAL CURRY

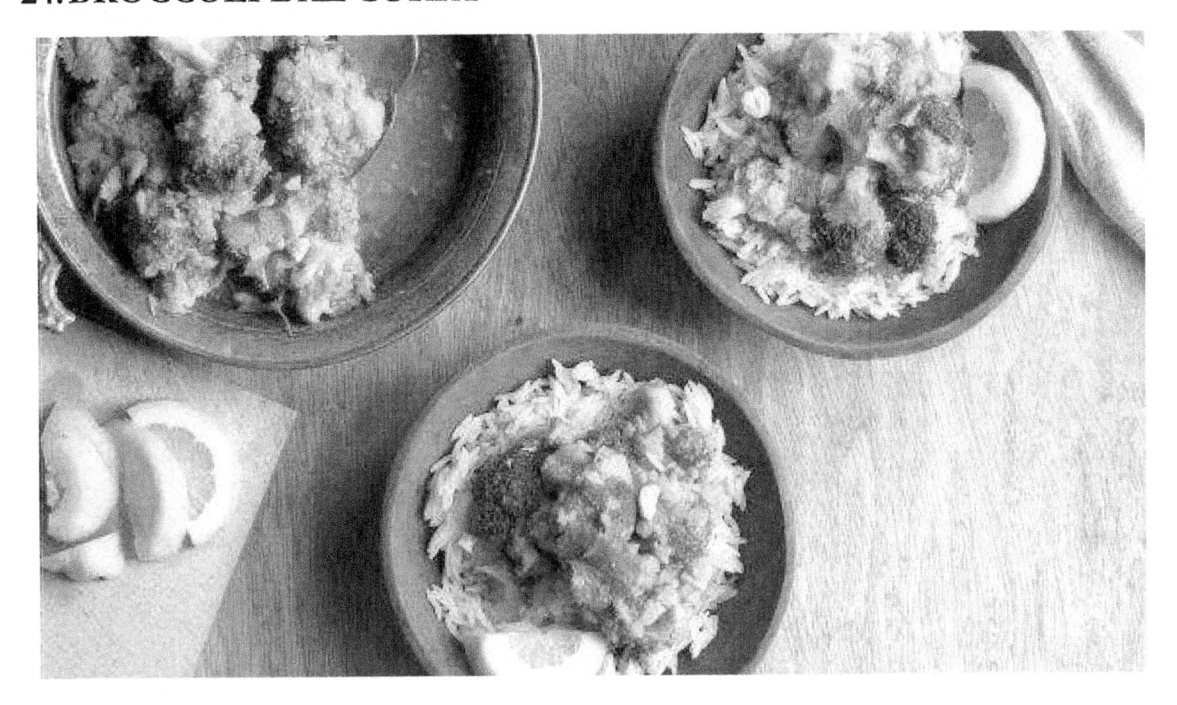

INGREDIENTS

- 4 tablespoons butter or 4 tablespoons ghee
- 2 medium onions, chopped
- 1 teaspoon chili powder
- 1 1/2 teaspoons black pepper
- 2 teaspoons cumin
- 1 teaspoon ground coriander
- 2 teaspoons turmeric
- 1 cup red lentil
- 1 lemon, juice of
- 3 cups chicken broth
- 2 medium broccoli, chopped
- ½ cup dried coconut (optional)
- 1 tablespoon flour
- 1 teaspoon salt
- 1 cup cashews, coarsely chopped (optional)

DIRECTIONS

- Heat butter in a saucepan and saute onions until well browned.

- Add chili powder, pepper, cumin, coriander, and turmeric.
- Stir and cook, 1 minute.
- Add lentils, lemon juice, broth, and coconut if using.
- Bring to boil, reduce heat and simmer for 45-55 minutes (if the mixture is too thick, you may need to add a little hot water).
- Steam broccoli for 7 minutes.
- Plunge broccoli in cold water and set it aside.
- Remove 1/3 cup of liquid from the lentil mixture.
- Add to flour to form a smooth paste.
- Return to pan; add broccoli, salt, and nuts if using.
- Simmer for 5 minutes.
- Serve over Basmati rice.

NUTRITION INFO

Serving Size: 1 (669) g

Servings Per Recipe: 4

- Calories: 445
- Calories from Fat 138 g
- Total Fat 15.4 g
- Saturated Fat 8 g
- Cholesterol 30.5 mg
- Sodium 1362.4 mg
- Total Carbohydrate 59 g
- Dietary Fiber 15.1 g
- Sugars 8.5 g
- Protein 25.7 g

25. SHEET PAN CHICKEN AND BRUSSEL SPROUTS

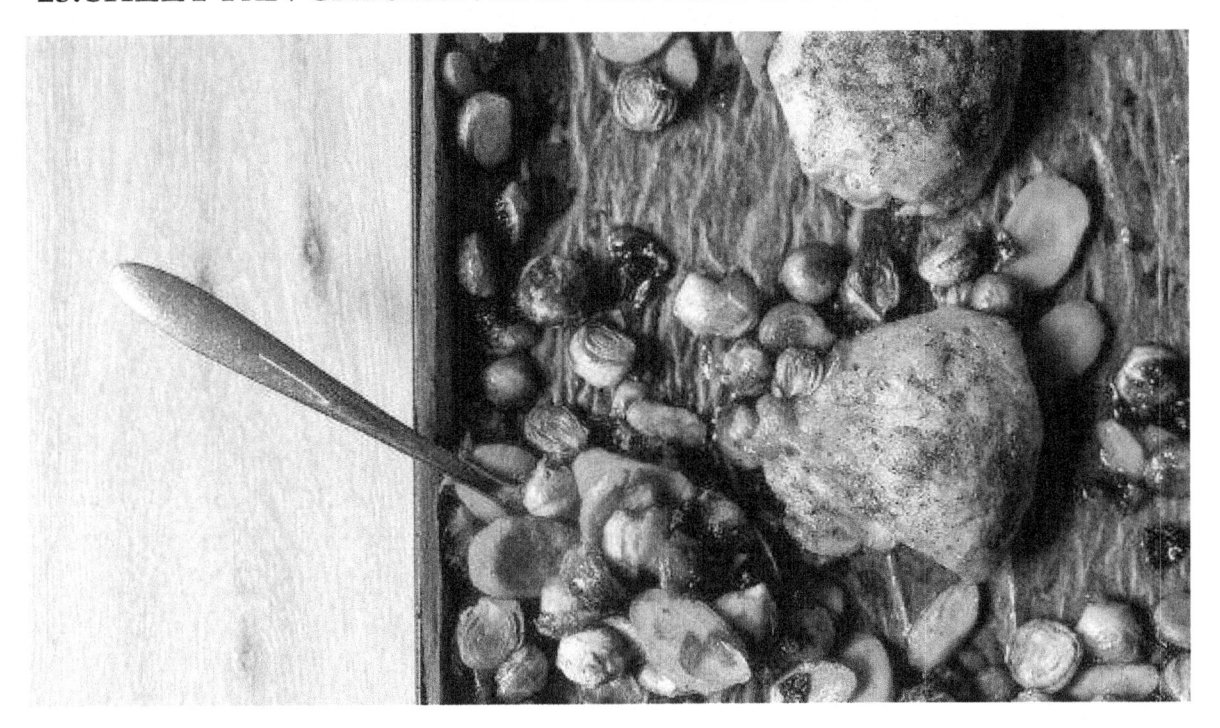

INGREDIENTS

- 4 skin-on chicken thighs
- 1 ½ cups Brussels sprouts, halved
- 4 carrots, cut on the bias
- 3 tablespoons olive oil
- 1 teaspoon herbes de Provence

DIRECTIONS

- Preheat oven to 400° F.
- Put cut vegetables into a bowl and add 1½ tbsp olive oil, ½ tsp herbs, and salt and pepper. Rub all over vegetables.
- Place veggies on a sheet pan.
- Add chicken thighs to the same bowl. Drizzle with 1½ tbsp olive oil, ½ tsp herbs, and salt and pepper. Rub all over the chicken.
- Place chicken on pan.
- Roast for; about 30-35 minutes or until chicken is done.
- If you prefer a crispier vegetable or chicken skin, turn the oven to broil and cook for a minute or two. Watch carefully or it will burn.

NUTRITION INFO

Serving Size: 1 (194) g

Servings Per Recipe: 4

- Calories: 323.4
- Calories from Fat 222 g
- Total Fat 24.8 g
- Saturated Fat 5.5 g
- Cholesterol 79 mg
- Sodium 119.9 mg
- Total Carbohydrate 7.9 g
- Dietary Fiber 2.5 g
- Sugars 3.4 g
- Protein 17.6 g

26. PERFECT CAULIFLOWER PIZZA CRUST

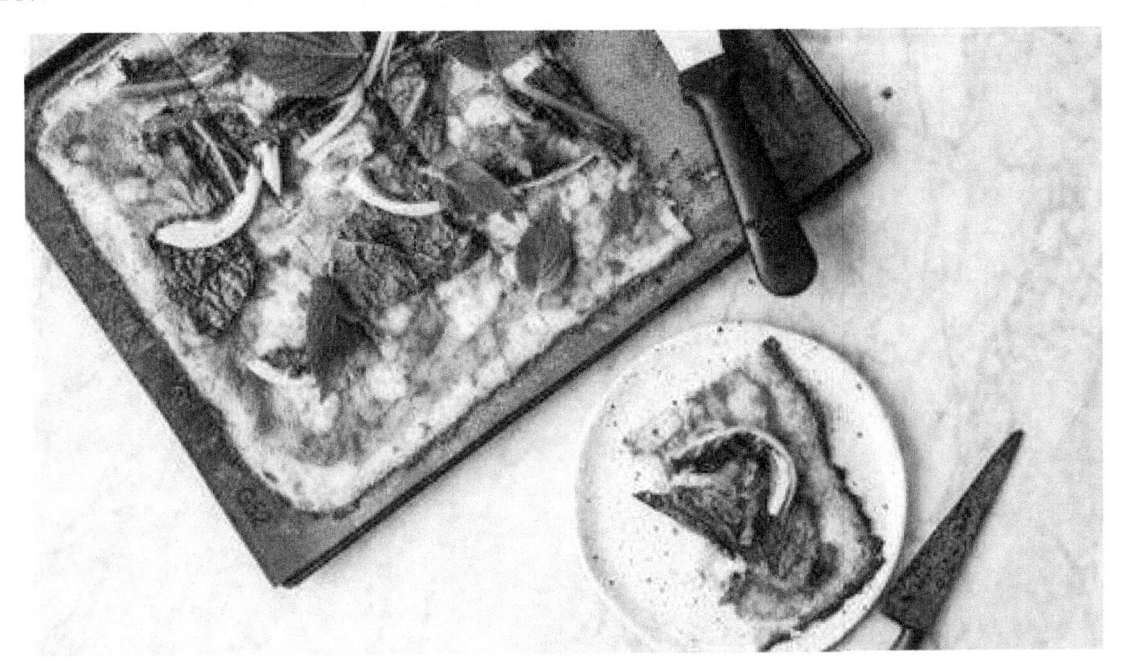

INGREDIENTS

- 1cups raw cauliflower, riced, or 1 medium cauliflower head
- egg, beaten
- 1 cup chevre cheese or 1 cup other soft cheese
- 1 teaspoon dried oregano
- 1 pinch salt

DIRECTIONS

- Preheat your oven to 400°F.
- To make the cauliflower rice, pulse batches of raw cauliflower florets in a food processor, until a rice-like texture is achieved.
- Fill a large pot with about an inch of water, and bring it to a boil. Add the "rice" and cover; let it cook for about 4-5 minutes. Drain into a fine-mesh strainer.
- THIS IS THE SECRET: Once you've strained the rice, transfer it to a clean, thin dishtowel. Wrap up the steamed rice in the dishtowel, twist it up, then SQUEEZE all the excess moisture out! It's amazing how much extra liquid will be released, which will leave you with a nice and dry pizza crust.
- In a large bowl, mix up your strained rice, beaten egg, goat cheese, and spices. (Don't be afraid to use your hands! You want it very well mixed.) It won't be like any pizza dough you've ever worked with, but don't worry– it'll hold together!

- Press the dough out onto a baking sheet lined with parchment paper. (It must be lined with parchment paper, or it will stick.) Keep the dough about 3/8" thick, and make the edges a little higher for a "crust" effect, if you like.
- Bake for 35-40 minutes at 400°F The crust should be firm, and golden brown when finished.
- Now's the time to add all your favorites– sauce, cheese, and any other toppings you like. Return the pizza to the 400F oven, and bake an additional 5-10 minutes, just until the cheese is hot and bubbly.
- Slice and serve immediately!

NUTRITION INFO

Serving Size: 1 (119) g

Servings Per Recipe: 4

- Calories: 45.3
- Calories from Fat 13 g
- Total Fat 1.5 g
- Saturated Fat 0.5 g
- Cholesterol 46.5 mg
- Sodium 88.7 mg
- Total Carbohydrate 5.6 g
- Dietary Fiber 2.2 g
- Sugars 2.1 g
- Protein 3.6 g

27. SWEET POTATO AND BLACK BEAN BURRITO

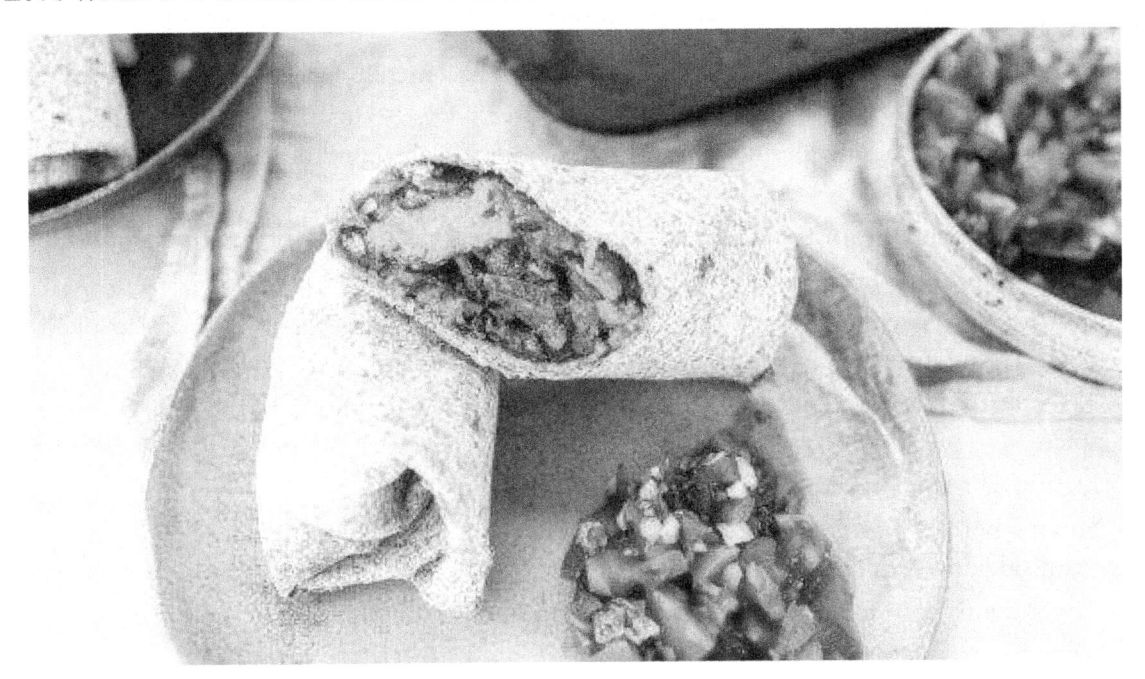

INGREDIENTS

- 1/2 cups peeled cubed sweet potatoes
- 2 teaspoon salt
- 2 teaspoons other vegetable oil or 2 teaspoons broth
- 3 1/2 cups diced onions
- 4 garlic cloves, minced (or pressed)
- 1 tablespoon minced fresh green chili pepper
- 4 teaspoons ground cumin
- 4 teaspoons ground coriander
- 4 1/2 cups cooked black beans (three 15-ounce cans, drained)
- 2/3 cup lightly packed cilantro leaf
- 2 tablespoons fresh lemon juice
- 1 teaspoon salt
- 12 (10 inches) flour tortillas
- fresh salsa

DIRECTIONS

- Preheat the oven to 350.
- Place the sweet potatoes in a medium saucepan with salt and water to cover.

- Cover and bring to a boil, then simmer until tender, about 10 minutes.
- Drain and set aside.
- While the sweet potatoes are cooking, warm the oil in a medium skillet or saucepan and add the onions, garlic, and chile.
- Cover and cook on medium-low heat, stirring occasionally, until the onions are tender, about 7 minutes.
- Add the cumin and coriander and cook for 2 to 3 minutes longer, stirring frequently.
- Remove from the heat and set aside.
- In a food processor, combine the black beans, cilantro, lemon juice, salt, and cooked sweet potatoes and puree until smooth (or mash the ingredients in a large bowl by hand).
- Transfer the sweet potato mixture to a large mixing bowl and mix in the cooked onions and spices.
- Lightly oil a large baking dish.
- Spoon about 2/3 to 3/4 cup of the filling in the center of each tortilla, roll it up, and place it, seam side down, in the baking dish.
- Cover tightly with foil and bake for about 30 minutes, until piping hot.
- Serve topped with salsa.

NUTRITION INFO

Serving Size: 1 (2933) g

Servings Per Recipe: 1

- Calories: 575.2
- Calories from Fat 92 g
- Total Fat 10.3 g
- Saturated Fat 2.3 g
- Cholesterol 0 mg
- Sodium 1156.4 mg
- Total Carbohydrate 102 g
- Dietary Fiber 15.9 g
- Sugars 8.7 g
- Protein 19.8 g

28. CROCKPOT BLACK EYED PEAS

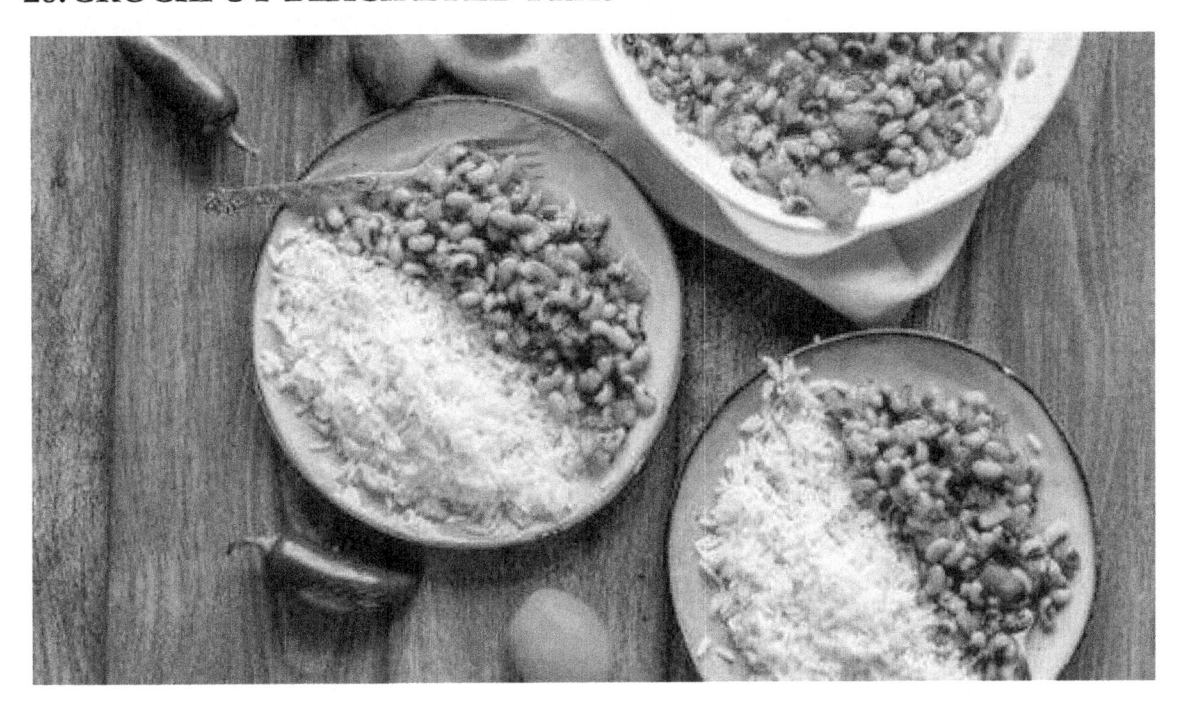

INGREDIENTS

- (16 ounces) bag dried black-eyed peas
- 1 small ham hock
- 1 (14 1/2 ounce) can Del Monte zesty jalapeno pepper diced tomato
- 1 (14 1/2 ounce) can diced tomatoes with green chilies
- 2 (10 1/2 ounce) can chicken broth
- 1 stalk celery, chopped

DIRECTIONS

- Pre-soak black-eyed peas according to the instructions on the bag.
- Combine all ingredients and cook on low for 9-10 hours.

NUTRITION INFO

Serving Size: 1 (257) g

Servings Per Recipe: 6

- Calories: 282.5
- Calories from Fat 14 g

- Total Fat 1.6 g
- Saturated Fat 0.4 g
- Cholesterol 0 mg
- Sodium 618.8 mg
- Total Carbohydrate 48.5 g
- Dietary Fiber 8.1 g
- Sugars 5.7 g
- Protein 20.5 g

29. PEACH BERRY SMOOTHIE

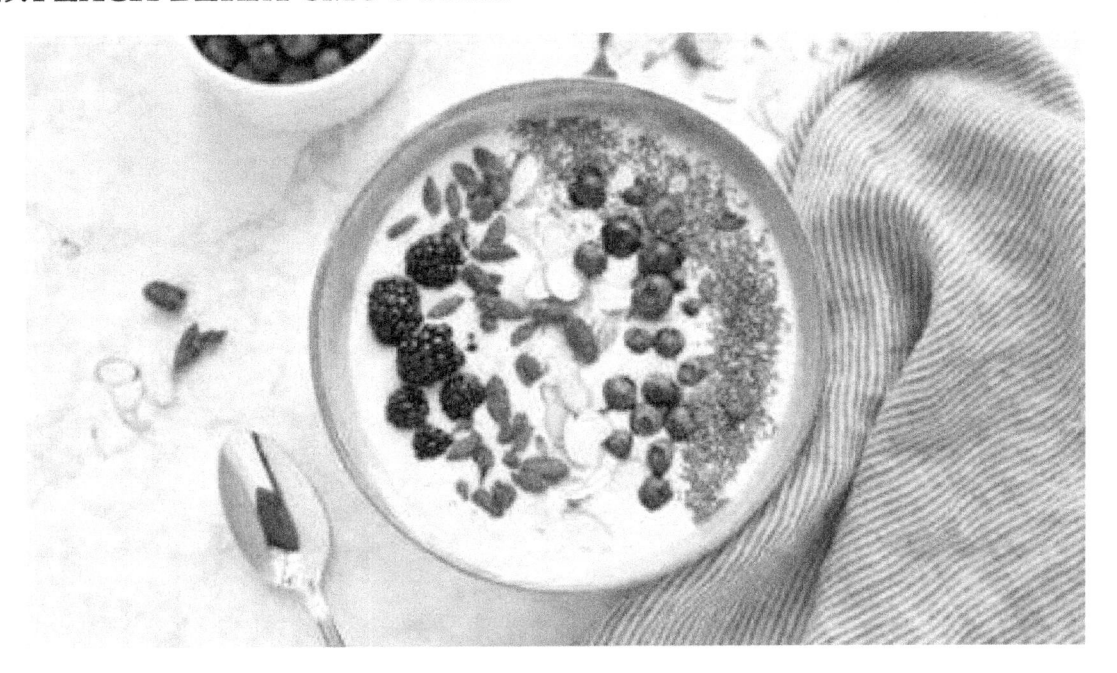

INGREDIENTS

- 1 cup frozen peaches
- ¼ cup coconut milk (adjust for a thicker or thinner smoothie)
- ½ cup Greek yogurt
- ½ teaspoon almond flavoring

DIRECTIONS

- Mix peaches through almond flavoring in a high-speed blender.
- Check the thickness and adjust accordingly. Add more milk for thinner and more peaches for thicker.
- Top with gorgeous toppings like chia seeds, berries, and slivered almonds.
- Enjoy.

NUTRITION INFO

Serving Size: 1 (308) g

Servings Per Recipe: 1

- Calories: 351.3
- Calories from Fat 111 g

- Total Fat 12.4 g
- Saturated Fat 10.7 g
- Cholesterol 0 mg
- Sodium 22.4 mg
- Total Carbohydrate 61.6 g
- Dietary Fiber 4.5 g
- Sugars 55.5 g
- Protein 2.7 g

30. SWEET POTATO CURRY WITH SPINACH AND CHICKPEAS

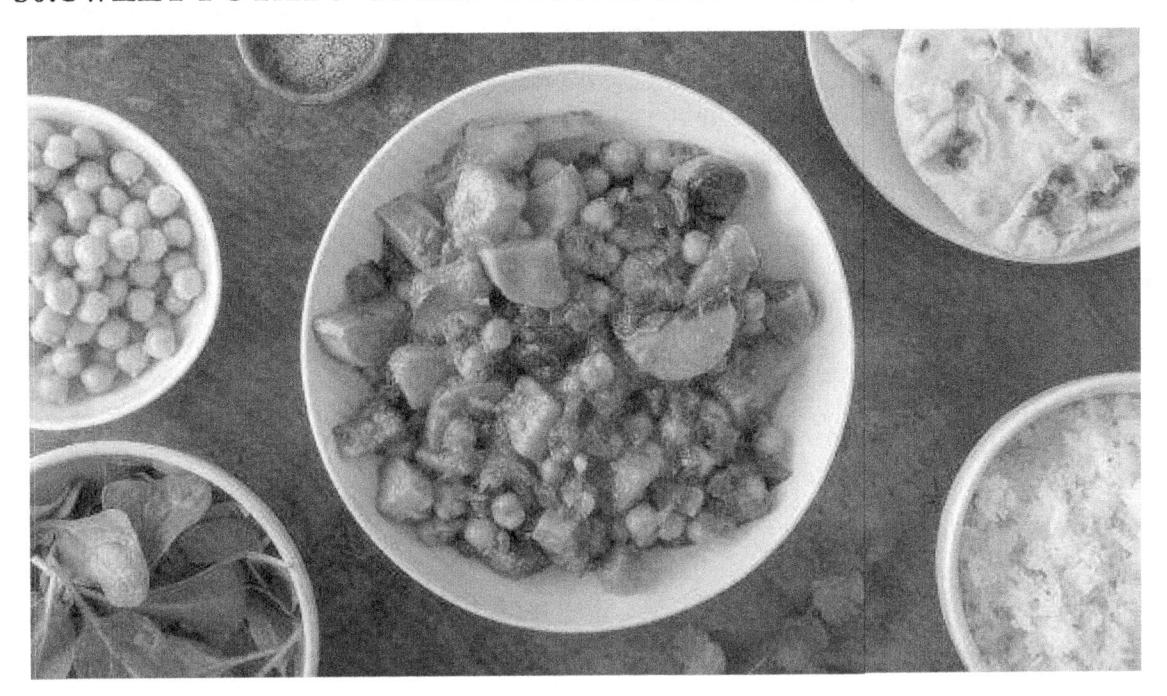

INGREDIENTS

- 1/2 large sweet onions, chopped or 2 scallions, thinly sliced
- 1 -2 teaspoon canola oil
- 2 tablespoons curry powder
- 1 tablespoon cumin
- 1 teaspoon cinnamon
- 10 ounces fresh spinach, washed, stemmed, and coarsely chopped
- 2 large sweet potatoes, peeled and diced (about 2 lbs)
- 1 (14 1/2 ounce) can chickpeas, rinsed and drained
- 1/2 cup water
- 1 (14 1/2 ounce) can diced tomatoes, can substitute fresh if available
- 1/4 cup chopped fresh cilantro, for garnish
- basmati rice or brown rice, for serving

DIRECTIONS

- You may choose to cook the sweet potatoes however you prefer.
- I like to peel, chop and steam mine in a veggie steamer for about 15 minutes.
- Baking or boiling work well too.
- While sweet potatoes cook, heat 1-2 tsp of canola or vegetable oil over medium heat.

- Add onions and sauté 2-3 minutes, or until they begin to soften.
- Next, add the curry powder, cumin, and cinnamon, and stir to coat the onions evenly with spices.
- Add tomatoes with their juices, and the chickpeas, stir to combine.
- Add ½ cup water and raise heat up to a strong simmer for about a minute or two.
- Next, add the fresh spinach, a couple of handfuls at a time, stirring to coat with cooking liquid.
- When all the spinach is added to the pan, cover and simmer until just wilted, about 3 minutes.
- Add the cooked sweet potatoes to the liquid, and stir to coat.
- Simmer for another 3-5 minutes, or until flavors are well combined.
- Transfer to serving dish, toss with fresh cilantro and serve hot.
- This dish is nice served over basmati or brown rice

NUTRITION INFO

Serving Size: 1 (269) g

Servings Per Recipe: 6

- Calories: 166.5
- Calories from Fat 21 g
- Total Fat 2.4 g
- Saturated Fat 0.3 g
- Cholesterol 0 mg
- Sodium 277.5 mg
- Total Carbohydrate 32 g
- Dietary Fiber 7.5 g
- Sugars 4.5 g
- Protein 6.8 g

31. POACHED EGGS & AVOCADO TOASTS

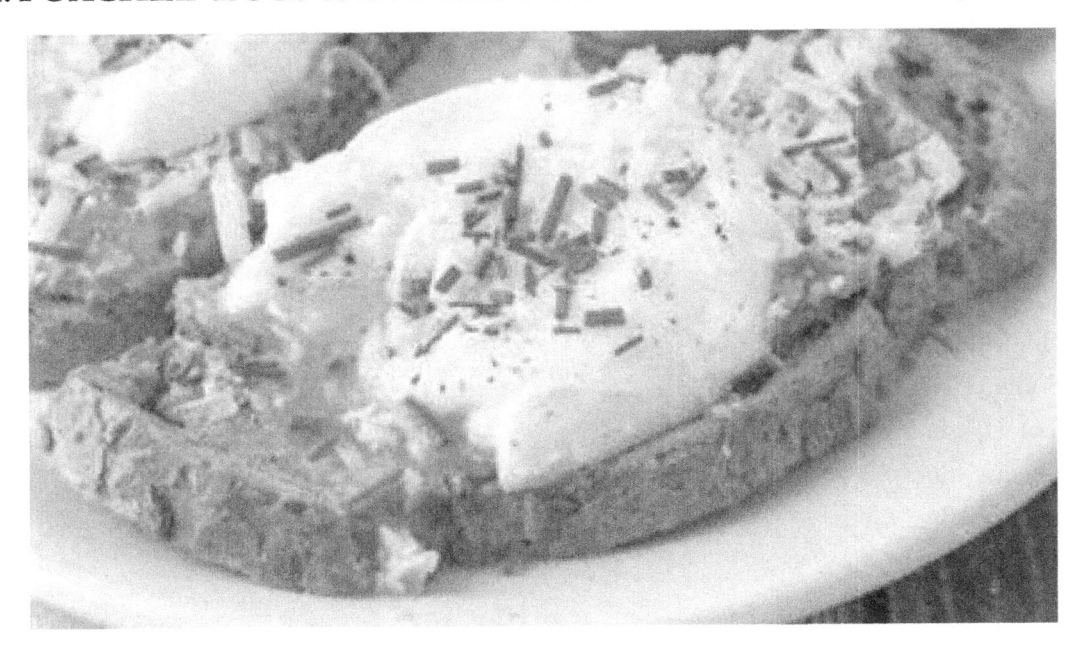

INGREDIENTS

- 4 eggs
- 2 ripe avocados
- 2 teaspoons lemon juice (or juice of 1 lime)
- 4 slices thick bread
- 1 cup cheese (grated, edam, gruyere, or whatever you have on hand)
- salt & freshly ground black pepper
- 4 teaspoons butter (for spreading on toast)

DIRECTIONS

- Poach eggs using your favorite method.
- Meanwhile cut the avocados in half and remove the stones.
- Using a spoon scoop out the flesh into a bowl and add the lemon or lime juice and the salt & pepper.
- Mash roughly using a fork.
- Toast the bread and spread it with butter.
- Spread the avocado mix onto each slice of buttered toast and top each with a poached egg.
- Sprinkle over the grated cheese and serve immediately.
- These are also nice with either fresh or grilled tomato halves on the side.

NUTRITION INFO

Serving Size: 1 (216) g

Servings Per Recipe: 4

- Calories: 439.8
- Calories from Fat 280 g
- Total Fat 31.2 g
- Saturated Fat 10.7 g
- Cholesterol 214.2 mg
- Sodium 537.7 mg
- Total Carbohydrate 26.6 g
- Dietary Fiber 7.5 g
- Sugars 2.2 g
- Protein 16.2 g

32. FRENCH VANILLA ALMOND GRANOLA

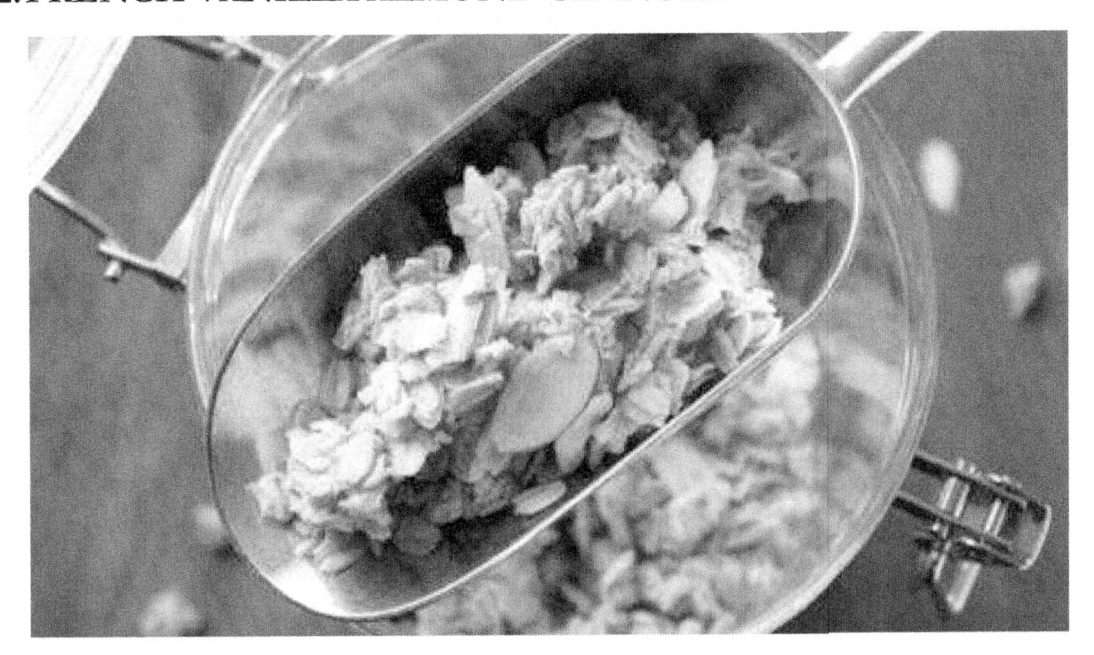

INGREDIENTS

- 3 1/2 cups old fashioned oats (not quick)
- 1/2 cup sliced almonds
- 1/2 cup water
- 1/2 cup natural cane sugar
- 1/4 teaspoon salt
- 1/4 cup organic canola oil or 1/4 cup grapeseed oil
- 1 tablespoon vanilla extract

DIRECTIONS

- Heat oven to 200 degrees F. Line a large, rimmed cookie sheet with parchment paper.
- In a large bowl mix together the oats and almonds.
- In a small saucepan over medium heat, stir the sugar and salt into the water. Cook and stir until sugar is dissolved. Remove from heat. Stir in canola oil and vanilla. Pour into the oat and almond mixture and stir until thoroughly combined.
- Spread mixture out on the lined cookie sheet and bake for 2 hours, or until dry to the touch. Do not stir! Remove from oven and let cool before breaking apart into chunks. Store in an airtight container.

NUTRITION INFO

Serving Size: 1 (51) g

Servings Per Recipe: 12

- Calories: 187.1
- Calories from Fat 71 g
- Total Fat 8 g
- Saturated Fat 0.7 g
- Cholesterol 0 mg
- Sodium 50.4 mg
- Total Carbohydrate 25.3 g
- Dietary Fiber 2.9 g
- Sugars 8.8 g
- Protein 3.9 g

33. MILLET & QUINOA MEDITERRANEAN SALAD

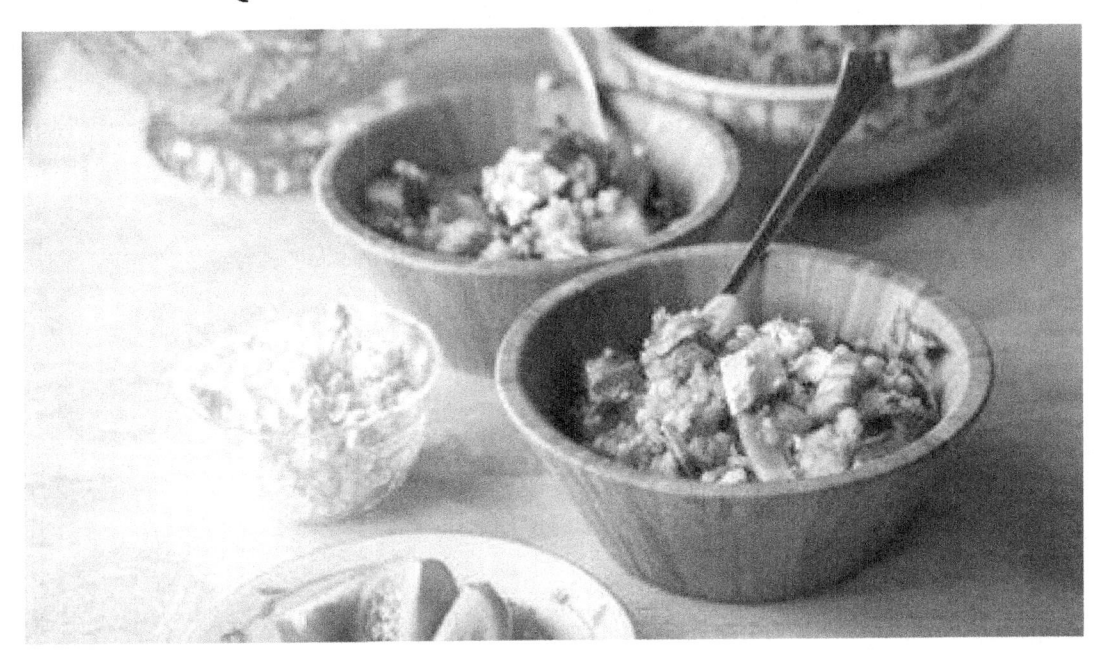

INGREDIENTS

- 1/2 cup millet
- 1 cup water
- 1/2 cup quinoa (red, white, or black)
- 3/4 cup water
- 1 English cucumber, diced
- 1 tomato, ripe, seeds squeezed out, diced
- 1 sweet pepper, seeded, diced
- 1/2 red onion, sliced thin
- 1 garlic clove, pressed
- 200g feta cheese, diced
- 1 (10 ounces) can large white beans, drained
- 1/4 teaspoon cayenne pepper (more, to taste)
- 2 teaspoons dried dill (sub basil or oregano, if preferred)
- 1/4 cup pine nuts
- 1 lemon, juice of (zest as well, if preferred)
- 1 tablespoon olive oil (optional)
- fresh ground pepper, to taste

DIRECTIONS

- Bring millet and 1 cup water to boil, reduce heat, and simmer for five minutes; turn off heat, cover, and let sit for 10 minutes.
- Bring quinoa and 3/4 cup water to boil, reduce heat, and simmer, covered, for 12-14 minutes; fluff.
- Combine all ingredients and toss; chill. Enjoy!

NUTRITION INFO

Serving Size: 1 (448) g

Servings Per Recipe: 3

- Calories: 641
- Calories from Fat 231 g
- Total Fat 25.7 g
- Saturated Fat 11.1 g
- Cholesterol 59.3 mg
- Sodium 764.6 mg
- Total Carbohydrate 78.6 g
- Dietary Fiber 12.6 g
- Sugars 9.1 g
- Protein 27.6 g

Conclusion

Intermittent fasting is simple to enforce since it does not necessitate calorie restriction or adherence to a strict diet but simply requires you to avoid eating for a period of time. The 16/8 rhythm is the most common and simple method: fasting at 4 p.m., eating at 8 p.m. You must pay attention to the carbohydrates in your day if you want to achieve faster results, whether it's losing weight or enhancing your efficiency. As a result, intermittent fasting will make getting into ketosis much easier.

Made in the USA
Middletown, DE
04 May 2021